P9-CFF-445

SCHENECTADY CO PUBLIC LIBRARY

THE REAL

SKINNY

DISCARDED

APPETITE FOR HEALTH'S 101
FAT HABITS & SLIM SOLUTIONS

Julie Upton, M.S., R.D., CSSD
& Katherine Brooking, M.S., R.D.

JEREMY P. TARCHER/PENGUIN
a member of Penguin Group (USA) Inc.
New York

JEREMY P. TARCHER/PENGUIN
Published by the Penguin Group
Penguin Group (USA) Inc., 375 Hudson Street,
New York, New York 10014, USA

USA · Canada · UK · Ireland · Australia
New Zealand · India · South Africa · China

Penguin Books Ltd, Registered Offices:
80 Strand, London WC2R 0RL, England
For more information about the Penguin Group visit penguin.com

Copyright © 2013 by Julie Upton & Katherine Brooking
All rights reserved. No part of this book may be reproduced, scanned,
or distributed in any printed or electronic form without permission.
Please do not participate in or encourage piracy of copyrighted materials in
violation of the authors' rights. Purchase only authorized editions.
Published simultaneously in Canada

Most Tarcher/Penguin books are available at special quantity discounts for bulk purchase for sales
promotions, premiums, fund-raising, and educational needs. Special books or book excerpts
also can be created to fit specific needs. For details, write Penguin Group (USA) Inc.
Special Markets, 375 Hudson Street, New York, NY 10014.

Library of Congress Cataloging-in-Publication Data

Upton, Julie, date.
The real skinny : appetite for health's 101 fat habits & slim solutions /
Julie Upton, M.S., R.D., CSSD, & Katherine Brooking, M.S., R.D.
p.   cm.
Includes bibliographical references and index.
ISBN 978-0-399-16382-1
1. Reducing diets—Recipes—Popular works.   2. Weight loss—Popular works.
3. Nutrition—Popular works.   I. Brooking, Katherine.   II. Title.
RM222.2.U68   2013   2012050284
613.2'5—dc23

Printed in the United States of America
1   3   5   7   9   10   8   6   4   2

BOOK DESIGN BY TANYA MAIBORODA

Neither the publisher nor the authors are engaged in rendering professional advice or services to the
individual reader. The ideas, procedures, and suggestions contained in this book are not intended
as a substitute for consulting with your physician. All matters regarding your health require
medical supervision. Neither the authors nor the publisher shall be liable or responsible for
any loss or damage allegedly arising from any information or suggestion in this book.

CONTENTS

INTRODUCTION:
THE REAL SKINNY ON
THE HABITS THAT MAKE US FAT

WHEN YOU LIVE IN THE UNITED STATES, FAT HAPPENS—EASILY. IF you are struggling to lose weight or maintain a healthy weight, you're not alone. Nearly 70 percent of American adults are either overweight or obese. And it's little wonder: There are literally hundreds of factors that influence what, when, and how much we eat and drink every day.

Our genes influence us, as do the government, the environment, and city planners. The food industry, your parents' eating habits, portion sizes and packaging, education, social circles, spouse, work, finances, age, and sex can also tip the scale in the wrong direction. Before you even know what hit you, you might find yourself stuck with dozens of what we call "Fat Habits"—those daily unhealthy behaviors, choices, and actions that are keeping you out of your "skinny jeans."

Studies show that you make around two hundred food choices every day. Think about it: Do I want OJ with my Kashi or Special K, Starbucks or Peet's, sugar or Splenda, chips or an apple, grilled chicken or Tex-Mex, an extra helping of rice, or cookies or a piece of cake while watching *Modern Family*?

Your weight is a reflection of the sum of all your daily habits, and with so many of us being overweight or obese, most of us need to know how to tone up and slim down our Fat Habits. That's why we wrote this book: We want *you* to be armed with all the information and tools you need to successfully navigate the complex world of food. When your everyday choices are good, it's easy to keep your weight in check. When your habits pile on extra calories from low-quality food choices that are rich in added sugars or saturated fat, pounds pile on.

As nutritionists, we know that there's nothing simple about losing weight and keeping it off. That's why half of all adults are on a diet right now. Millions are probably going off those diets just as you're reading this sentence. Most dieters lose steam because the diets they're on don't fit their lifestyle or are too restrictive, or they let a slipup derail all their efforts. As a result, few are successful at losing significant amounts of weight and keeping it off when following a typical "diet."

Our approach is completely different, because we take a nondiet approach that focuses on progress, not perfection, and simple changes that add up to pounds off. Going on a diet that focuses on eliminating problem foods, such as wheat-free plans, or paleo approaches that make entire food groups off-limits, is setting yourself up for failure. As a rule, if you can't stick with something for life, it's not likely to work.

The good news is that despite all of the minefields that can lead to extra pudge, you have the power to prevail over stumbling blocks, setbacks, and saboteurs that inhibit you from reaching your goals. You can take charge of your weight fate. And we're going to help you succeed!

WHAT MAKES *THE REAL SKINNY* DIFFERENT

First, this isn't a diet book. It's a tool that we want you to use daily to make positive behavior changes in your life. We believe and promote healthy eating of wholesome, quality foods, the foods you love and crave, but doing so in ways that allow you to enjoy a fit, healthy body and life. We focus on eating healthy foods combined with functional fitness. If your diet is full of delicious, great-tasting, high-quality choices, you won't necessarily have to count calories to achieve weight loss.

We wrote *The Real Skinny: Appetite for Health's 101 Fat Habits and Slim Solutions* based on what we heard from the hundreds of thousands of fans who visit our website, Appetite for Health (AppforHealth.com), where we share what we eat and provide daily diet and nutrition advice.

Our readers sent us comments complaining about how they had gained weight and just couldn't seem to get it to budge. Most were repeat dieters who had tried everything from celebrity-endorsed diets to detox diets, commercial weight-loss programs, and more. Like other frustrated dieters, they were spending oodles of money on diet pills, powders, books, and plans that didn't address the underlying habits that ultimately derailed their efforts to reach a healthy weight.

By helping our fans find solutions for their weight woes, we identified many common habits people face when dieting. It's from our conversations with our readers that we compiled the 101 worst Fat Habits. Luckily, from our work with fans, many of whom were able to take control over their diet and eating, we proved that healthy eating is delicious, satisfying, and *always* possible—no matter the circumstances.

PUTTING THE SCIENCE INTO PRACTICE . . . ON YOUR PLATE

As registered dietitians, we've spent years studying human nutrition and even have graduate degrees in nutrition science. Together we've helped thousands of people and have more than thirty years of experience in nutrition.

As nutrition professionals, all of our recommendations are based on significant scientific agreement. To write this book, we combed through thousands of weight-loss studies to look at the major reasons why so many of us are overweight. We looked at biological, psychological, neurological, behavioral, and social science studies to give us comprehensive solutions to treat overweight from every angle.

We were able to "digest" the results of those studies to provide our Slim Solutions for everyday living. We give you the practical tools and tricks to combat the current behaviors that are standing between you and your healthy weight goals. Everything from the temperature of your house to your office environment, your daily screen time, emotional triggers, and foods that hijack your body's hunger hormones is considered in each of our recommendations.

When you identify your Fat Habits and replace them with Slim Solutions, you'll lose weight—period. This is the foundation of *The Real Skinny: Appetite for Health's 101 Fat Habits and Slim Solutions.*

Let's face it: Diets equal deprivation. Think of us as diet centrists. We don't provide a diet prescription, like wheat-free, low fat, vegan, high protein, or low carb. We're about healthy living and positive behaviors that you can use and keep for life. We promote progress, not perfection. We help you identify and break your Fat Habits by giving you healthier Slim Solutions. Losing weight and

A Word About Fat

We realize that the F-word—"fat"—is usually emotionally charged. Many people associate the word "fat" with being teased as a chubby child, or as the source of low self-esteem at any stage of life. And being called fat is certainly not a compliment in contemporary society. In the context of this book, however, we are reappropriating the word "fat." We mean "fat" simply as those extra pounds that are unhealthy. Our goal for you is not to be too slim, or even skinny; rather, it's for you to achieve optimal health in both body and mind, regardless of what the scale says. We believe healthy is the new skinny.

maintaining a healthy weight aren't always easy, but they are certainly doable. We're here to help make sure that happens.

Here's a look at what you can expect to learn in the following pages:

* Ways to identify Fat Habits that you have in your everyday life and empower yourself to overcome your barriers to losing weight and keeping it off for good.
* How to work with your food cravings so you can satisfy them without losing control.
* How to fool yourself full on fewer calories by tricking your hunger hormones with sleep, serving utensils, the time you eat, and various combinations of foods.
* Ways those with "fat genes" can learn to live and fit into skinny jeans. If you inherited genes that make gaining weight easy and losing hard, have a medical condition that makes it hard for you

The Skinny on Julie

There's nothing pleasant about being "pleasantly plump." I know because I was a fat kid. I was picked on, and I had to wear clothes from the "chubby" department, and my nickname was "Pickles" . . . and not because I liked them. I can vividly remember years of feeling embarrassed and uncomfortable in my own skin.

Despite having genes that make it easy for me to pile on pounds, I was fortunate that even though I was overweight, I had natural athletic ability. When I started to have more success in swimming, softball, and track and field, I immediately learned the connection between what I ate and my performance. When I started making simple substitutions for what I was eating, I lost nearly twenty pounds, so that by the time I graduated high school, I was physically fit, lean, and confident.

Because eating right changed my life outlook, I became a registered dietitian. And despite my family history of bad genes and my tendencies to "feed" my emotions, I've been able to maintain a healthy weight for more than twenty years. At the same time, I've been able to help others improve their eating and lifestyle habits to find their own success.

Like me, you may have a Fat Habit like bad genes that makes it hard to maintain a healthy weight. But this book provides the way to live lean despite your genes, or any other reason you're struggling with your weight.

■

to lose weight, or you're feeling older and pounds don't seem to come off like they once did, we'll provide novel Slim Solutions. We won't let overweight be your destiny.

- How to identify the skinnier menu choices when eating out—from four-star restaurants to fast-food joints.

- How a 1,600-calorie-a-day, fourteen-day meal plan gives you added structure and the template for healthy eating with the

The Skinny on Katherine

I guess you could say I lucked out when they were handing out a "weight DNA," because I did end up with a "skinny gene." But you don't have to be fat to have Fat Habits!

This I know firsthand: I began my career far from the field of nutrition and health, jumping right into the frenzied world of finance straight after college. Impossibly tight deadlines, stress, and ninety-hour workweeks were all too common. Before long I found myself living off greasy take-out food and dropping all of my favorite physical activities. It seemed that there just wasn't enough time to do my job well, maintain a social life, eat right, *and* stay fit.

It didn't take long for my unhealthy lifestyle to catch up with me. At the age of twenty-three, just two years after starting my career, I was out of energy and feeling completely unmotivated. Not only had I compromised my physical health, but I was most certainly *less* effective in my job. Even worse, I simply wasn't enjoying life.

That's when I decided something had to change. I began paying attention to what I ate and started doing yoga and Pilates. Ultimately the difference that this made in my life was so great I decided that I wanted to make healthy living—and teaching others how to preserve their health—my life's work. I left my Wall Street job and returned to school to pursue a master's in nutrition science and become a registered dietitian. After I earned my degrees, I began helping those who were struggling to make their own health a priority in their lives. My clients have included medical students, working moms, CEOs, and people from all walks of life looking to lose weight, boost their health, or just to feel more energized. I hope that this book will make you not only healthier but also happier with your body and your relationship with wholesome food.

exact number of servings you need daily from each of the food groups.

- Ways to look at how your family, friends, and colleagues impact your weight, and how to communicate your needs without "unfriending" anyone.

- How to shop for, prepare, and love wholesome, delicious food choices, like fresh fruits and veggies, lean proteins that help fill you up and not out, healthy fats that enhance the satisfaction of your meals and snacks, and satisfying whole grains.

- How to get over slipups, setbacks, or out-and-out pig-outs. Everyone messes up; it's how you get back on track that determines whether you will be successful at living slim.

- You'll get a taste of our thirty-three skinny recipes that fit into your meal plans and will help you gain more confidence in healthy cooking. Our recipes are made from simple, readily available ingredients and are quick and easy to make.

- We'll outline ways to fit more movement into your everyday life—no matter how time-pressed you are. Our ten-minute workouts focus on functional fitness using just your body weight to help you get fitter faster.

- You'll feel better, stronger, and more confident by swapping your Fat Habits for Slim Solutions.

THE REAL SKINNY

IT'S OUT OF MY CONTROL

"BECAUSE OF MY GENES, I CAN'T FIT INTO MY SKINNY JEANS!"

If you can rattle off a handful of excuses for why you're overweight—"I'm fifty years old"; "I inherited this body type"; "My parents never ate healthfully"; "I come from a family of nonathletes"—faster than you can recite your Social Security number, then you could very well be standing in the way of your own success. We know that there are many valid reasons why you may be overweight, but that said, they don't need to dictate whether or not you'll be successful at losing weight and keeping it off.

It's easier to blame someone or something else for our failures. After all, doing so allows us to ignore our role in the problem. If you believe your weight struggles are a result of bad genes or an unhealthy upbringing, then you don't have to look at the fact that what you do (eat too much) or don't do (exercise) every day is sabotaging your health and well-being.

Ready to put an end to the excuses once and for all? We're here to help. We'll show you how to empower yourself to overcome your unique barriers to losing weight and keeping it off for good. We don't want you to be a passive bystander in life; we want you to have the know-how and tools to create your healthy life—beginning now.

FAT HABIT #1

No matter what, I'm never going to lose weight—and I
don't think it's all my fault. —RACHEL M.

While the first part of that statement may be a slight exaggeration, the second part isn't totally unfounded. There's a lot of blame to go around when it comes to weight woes. We can point the finger at the food supply, your genes, your partner, your pals, local schools, the government, grocery stores, city planners, and more, and that's just for starters. The list is seemingly endless.

But don't give up hope. Identifying your particular weight-loss traps and knowing how to avoid or overcome them is key to shedding those extra pounds.

SLIM SOLUTIONS

MAKE A BLAME LIST

Jot down the name of every person or thing that contributes to your weight struggles. Then you can either decide to work on overcoming each of these "barriers" or simply accept them. Are we suggesting that you shouldn't even try? Absolutely not. We just know that part of being successful at losing weight is recognizing when you're truly ready to try. With planning, preparation, and practice, everyone can overcome their personal barriers and improve their diet and health.

TAKE THE QUIZ

Answer the following ten questions to see if you're really ready to lose weight.

ARE YOU READY TO LOSE?

1. | I've thought a lot about my eating habits and physical activities in order to pinpoint what I need to change.

True   *False*

2. | I've accepted the idea that I need to make permanent—not temporary—changes to be successful.

True   *False*

3. | I think losing weight slowly and safely would be preferable to losing it very quickly.

True   *False*

4. | I'm thinking about trying to lose weight because I really want to, not because someone else thinks I should.

True   *False*

5. | I'm willing and able to increase my physical activity.

True   *False*

6. | I'm at a stable point in my life where I can commit to weight loss and not get depressed by temporary setbacks, if they arise.

True   *False*

7. | I don't need to be "model thin" to consider my weight loss successful.

True   *False*

8. | I understand my likes and dislikes, and what makes me overeat.

True   *False*

9. | I am ready to eat differently even if it hurts my family's or my friends' feelings, or causes conflict.

True   *False*

10. | I'm willing to read this book and use the information provided to create a healthier diet and lifestyle.

True   *False*

If you answered "true" to seven or more of the questions above, you're ready to make the lifestyle changes that will help you lose weight. If you responded "false" to four or more questions, you may be contemplating change, but you haven't committed to it just yet. Keep reading—you may just find the inspiration to do so in these pages.

FAT HABIT #2

I have such a slow metabolism. I hardly eat anything
but just can't lose weight. —CAROL S.

Metabolism has spurred more urban legends than Bigfoot! The truth is, for more than 95 percent of us, our metabolic rate—the rate at which we burn calories—has nothing to do with our weight woes. In fact, numerous studies show that metabolism is inherently linked to body weight, and the more you weigh, the higher your metabolism. Most overweight people automatically believe that they have a "slow" metabolism, while the truth is, their metabolism is actually higher than those of their pin-thin friends.

And yet, if you Google the word "metabolism," you'll get more than 85 million hits, mostly on how to "speed up," "ignite," "kick-start," or "boost" your metabolism to blast fat and build muscle—and, of course, you can do all of this without cutting a single calorie.

Basal metabolic rate (BMR) represents the energy your body needs to sustain itself at rest and includes things like the energy cost of your heartbeat and breathing. (It does not count any activity.) For most women of average height and build, BMR is equal to .9 calories per kilogram of body weight per hour. That means a 130-pound woman would burn 1,300 calories in a day just to maintain all her body's functions. (A man's basal metabolic rate is

about 1 calorie/kg body weight per hour; men have a higher percentage of lean mass naturally compared with women, and thus have a higher basal metabolic rate.)

SLIM SOLUTIONS

FIGURE OUT YOUR METABOLIC RATE

You can use the easy metabolic rate equation above or the gold-standard Harris Benedict Equation below. There are also hundreds of metabolic rate calculators on the Internet, so you don't even have to get out your calculator.

What's Your Metabolic Rate?

Women: BMR = 655 + (9.6 × your weight in kg) + (1.8 × your height in cm) − (4.7 × your age in years)

Men: BMR = 66 + (13.7 × your weight in kg) + (5 × your height in cm) − (6.8 × your age in years)

[Note: 1 inch = 2.54 cm; 1 kilogram = 2.2 lbs]

FOR EXAMPLE:

You are female

You weigh 160 pounds (73 kilos)

You are 5 feet, 6 inches tall (167.6 cm)

You are 30 years old

Your BMR = 655 + 700 + 302 − 141 = **1,516 calories/day**

KNOW THE BMR BASICS

What affects your basal metabolic rate? Your age, sex, genes, body weight, diet, temperature, and altitude all impact the number of calories you burn in a day. Your organs—your brain, heart, liver, and kidneys—also help you burn calories. They require the most energy of all human tissues, but they make up a small percentage of our metabolic rate, because they're not major contributors to our total body weight. Muscles, on the other hand, contribute some 25 percent of your metabolic rate. That's a score for you, because you can significantly boost your muscle mass to increase your calorie burn.

BUILD A BIGGER CALORIE-BURNING ENGINE

You'd think being small would be a blessing. But what having a petite frame means is that your body naturally burns fewer calories because it doesn't require as much energy to maintain itself.

The Nutrition Twins (www.NutritionTwins.com), Lyssie Lakatos and Tammy Lakatos Shames, registered dietitians, personal trainers, and authors of *The Nutrition Twins' Veggie Cure* and *The Secret to Skinny*, know what it's like to have a small metabolic engine, because they're petite. As a result, they're always looking for ways to boost their naturally low metabolic rates, including:

- *Using interval training.* "As personal trainers, we always recommend doing high-intensity interval-type training to get the most out of your workouts. Interval training, which includes short bouts of high-intensity efforts with periods of active rest, has been shown to raise metabolism longer and higher than lower-intensity exercise. If you aren't working up a sweat during your workouts, it's not hard enough." See Chapter 8 for examples of our favorite interval workouts.
- *Staying well hydrated.* "Dehydration has been found to decrease your metabolic rate by two percent, so staying well hydrated is an easy way to help boost overall metabolic rate. Strive to get at least half of your body weight in fluid ounces of water every day. So if

you weigh 175 pounds, you should drink 87 ounces of water every day."

- *Pumping up your protein.* "The amount of energy the body requires to digest and metabolize food makes up only about 10 percent of your total metabolic rate. However, there are big differences in how many calories are burned during the digestion of each of the macronutrients. Fat, for example, has a thermic effect (a fancy term that simply refers to how much energy—aka calories—is expended during digestion and absorption) of 0 to 3 percent, carbohydrate is 5 to 10 percent, and protein is 20 to 30 percent.

   "That means when you eat 100 calories of protein, your body has to work to digest it—in the process, you might burn about 20 to 30 calories, leaving only 70 to 80 of the protein calories remaining for the body. Fat, on the other hand, requires barely any energy to digest, so if you were to consume 100 calories of fat, your body would be able to use or store all or most of them. Research shows that doubling your intake of protein from about 15 percent of calories to 30 percent of total calories can help you burn an extra 150 to 200 calories a day." That's why the menus we provide are higher in protein, to help your body burn calories more effortlessly.

- *Getting a caffeine fix.* "Caffeine can boost your metabolic rate for up to three hours after consumption. While you don't want to overdo caffeine, enjoying 3-4 cups of coffee or tea (especially green tea) daily can be a great way to get a little lift to your metabolism."

- *Building muscle.* "Muscles require more energy to maintain than fat tissue. What that means: The more muscle you have, the more calories your body naturally burns. For each pound of fat-free muscle mass you add to your frame, you'll boost your metabolic

Debunking a Major Metabolism Myth

Slim people have all the luck—good genes (and jeans) and a superfast metabolism. Believe it or not, heavier (and taller) people typically have a faster metabolism than thinner (and shorter) people. That's because the more weight you carry around, the more calories your body naturally burns to keep everything going. And the reverse is true: When you lose weight, your basal metabolic rate drops—your lighter body requires less energy to sustain itself at rest. That's partly why it's hard to maintain weight loss.

rate by 10 calories a day. Add five pounds of muscle, and you're up (or down!) an extra 50 calories a day. If that's not enough to get you galloping to your gym, there's one more benefit to building muscle: You'll get another metabolic boost from the muscle repair that happens in your body post-workout." (See our strength-training recommendations in Chapter 8.)

FAT HABIT #3

I'm addicted to all things sweet. —NINA B.

Your sweet tooth is a side effect of being human. We're programmed to like sweets—it's a survival mechanism that stems from our hunter-gatherer days, when we ate berries and other carbohydrate-rich plant foods that provided much-needed energy.

New brain chemistry research shows that certain foods, such as sugar and sugar-rich treats like chocolate, candy, and ice cream, stimulate areas of the brain that (A) make us feel good and (B) make us want more—a double diet whammy! And as with other types of addiction, the body craves more and more of the sugary stuff to get that same feel-good response.

This type of food neurochemistry research is still in its infancy, but investigators at Yale University found that some people are more susceptible to feeling "addicted" to certain foods or experiencing intense food cravings. These people are often overweight and tend to be more emotional in general and self-soothe with food.

If you can relate to being emotional, often use food to give yourself a lift, and are struggling with your weight, you may be someone who experiences food addiction–like symptoms.

SLIM SOLUTION

You can lick your sugar addiction once and for all. Julie did it, after she realized that she couldn't satisfy her sweet tooth despite the fact that she was using more and more sugar substitutes in her tea and coffee. She quit cold turkey two years ago and she's been able to stick to this for the most part (minus the premenstrual hormonal cravings she gets every month). Here's how she did it:

1. | *Can your soda habit.* Sodas and other sweetened beverages (including diet) provide about half of all the added sugar in the U.S. diet, so they're the first items you need to nix. They don't contribute to fullness, so you won't miss them—much.

2. | *Skip sugar substitutes.* These calorie-free sweeteners may actually trigger sweet cravings. They're hundreds of times sweeter than sugar—once you get accustomed to their intensity, it's hard to be satisfied with the natural sweetness of other foods.

3. | *Be a sugar sleuth.* For just one week, read the Nutrition Facts and ingredient list for everything you eat and drink. If a product contains more than 8 grams of "sugars" on the Nutrition

Facts panel, go directly to the ingredient list. If you see any form of added sugars (look for sucrose, dextrose, sorbitol, mannitol, honey, agave, dextrin, maltodextrin, high-fructose corn syrup, corn syrup, any syrup, anything ending with an "-ose" or "-ols"), skip it. If there is sugar listed on the Nutrition Facts panel but there is no sugar listed in the ingredient list, it means that the food or beverage contains natural sugars; don't worry about them, because they're not "metabolically equivalent" to added sugars.

4. | *Get off to a protein-rich start.* Begin your day with a protein-rich breakfast, like eggs with veggies, an egg-white omelet, or Greek yogurt with fruit. Research shows that people who eat breakfasts of eggs consumed 400 fewer calories over twenty-four hours compared with those who ate a more carb-heavy breakfast, like pancakes and waffles or toast with jam. Protein is known to be more filling and helps to regulate hunger hormones so that you stay fuller longer. (See our meal plans for protein-packed breakfasts.)

5. | *Go natural.* Focus on naturally sweet foods, like dried fruit, roasted veggies, and caramelized onions. There are many foods that provide natural sweetness—they've just been passed over for the more intensely sweet added sugars or sugar substitutes you've gotten used to.

After seven days of following a sugar-free eating plan, you can start experimenting with adding back limited amounts of sugars. Try to eat added sugars with other foods or at the end of a meal to minimize their effect on blood sugar and insulin levels. Like the American Heart Association, we recommend limiting added sugars to no more than 100 calories (or 6 teaspoons) a day. Use our meal plans to see how you can enjoy a sweet fix without consuming all those empty calories.

Drowning in the Sweet Stuff:
Not-So-Sweet Sugar Stats

- Americans eat about 22 teaspoons of added sugars a day. That's more than 70 pounds each year, with the majority coming from sugary beverages.
- A soda-a-day habit can add 30-plus pounds of added sugars to your diet in a year!
- The calories from nutrient-poor sweeteners add up to 128,480 calories per year.

FAT HABIT #4

I'm a curvy woman . . . we're supposed to be a little soft.

—CARRIE B.

While you may be thanking Jennifer Lopez, Beyoncé, and Kim Kardashian for making curves a commodity, beware: Most women underestimate how much body fat they have. We're not saying you shouldn't cherish your curvaceousness—just make sure that those "curves" aren't really extra pounds (which could increase your risk for breast cancer and heart disease and shorten your life) in disguise.

Women are biologically programmed to have five times more essential body fat than men. A woman needs 10 to 12 percent (whereas a man needs only 2 to 4 percent)—this extra body fat provides additional calories to help support a pregnancy and nursing. Men have higher levels of testosterone and other muscle-building hormones, which is why they have an easier time losing and maintaining a leaner body.

SLIM SOLUTIONS

GET MEASURED

Do you know what your body fat percentage is? If not, get it measured. Your goal: Between 20 and 31 percent is considered a "normal" range for most women, according to research. The ideal level for fitness (and looking fit) is around 20 to 22 percent, and topnotch female athletes generally have between 14 and 20 percent body fat. If you want to "see" your fab abs, don't worry about more crunches; just lower your body fat to about 18 to 20 percent.

There are many ways to measure body fat, from underwater weighing (which can be done at universities or at some health clubs) to body-fat calipers (the person should be well trained at taking measurements). If you prefer a more private measurement, you can get a bathroom scale that takes bioelectric impedance body-fat measurements. They're readily available and easy to use.

FIND YOUR HEALTHY WEIGHT

Everyone has a "healthy weight"—the number (or range, even) at which you feel great and your body is performing at its best. This number varies—even women of the same height and same shape may have very different healthy weights. Remember, body weight and body fat are impacted by your genetic background, how much you exercise, and, to some extent, how old you are.

What's your healthy weight? The Metropolitan Life heightweight tables, which were used for years to determine whether you were at an optimal weight, were replaced by the Body Mass Index as the standard medical professionals use to determine healthy weight or body fat measurements. Yet many professionals (us included) often think that BMI can be a bit too generous for women, and that's why we still like the old Metropolitan Life height-weight tables.

To begin, you'll need to know whether you have a small, medium, or large frame. Here's how you can tell:

Measure the circumference of your wrist.

IF YOU'RE UNDER 5 FEET, 2 INCHES

Small frame = wrist size less than 5½ inches

Medium frame = wrist size 5½ inches to 5¾ inches

Large frame = wrist size more than 5¾ inches

IF YOU'RE BETWEEN 5 FEET, 2 INCHES AND 5 FEET, 5 INCHES

Small frame = wrist size less than 6 inches

Medium frame = wrist size 6 inches to 6¼ inches

Large frame = wrist size more than 6¼ inches

IF YOU'RE OVER 5 FEET, 5 INCHES

Small frame = wrist size less than 6¼ inches

Medium = wrist size 6¼ inches to 6½ inches

Large = wrist size more than 6½ inches

Once you know your frame size, look at the charts on the following pages to find your height and ideal weight range.

CHECK YOUR WAIST CIRCUMFERENCE

Where you carry your weight can tip you off to potential problems in the future. For instance, if you tend to carry your weight in the middle (often referred to as an apple shape), you may be at increased risk for heart disease, type 2 diabetes, breast cancer, and other chronic conditions. But there's good news: The fat in your middle is easier to whittle away than the fat that resides in your hips and butt.

MEN			
HEIGHT FEET INCHES	SMALL FRAME	MEDIUM FRAME	LARGE FRAME
5' 2"	128–134	131–141	138–150
5' 3"	130–136	133–143	140–153
5' 4"	132–138	135–145	142–156
5' 5"	134–140	137–148	144–160
5' 6"	136–142	139–151	146–164
5' 7"	138–145	142–154	149–168
5' 8"	140–148	145–157	152–172
5' 9"	142–151	148–160	155–176
5' 10"	144–154	151–163	158–180
5' 11"	146–157	154–166	161–184
6' 0"	149–160	157–170	164–188
6' 1"	152–164	160–174	168–192
6' 2"	155–168	164–178	172–197
6' 3"	158–172	167–182	176–202
6' 4"	162–176	171–187	181–207

Weights at ages 25–59 based on lowest mortality. Weight in pounds according to frame (in indoor clothing weighing 5 lbs.; shoes with 1" heels).

TO MEASURE YOUR MIDDLE:

- Place a tape measure around your bare stomach, just above your hip bone.
- Pull the tape measure until it fits snugly around you, but doesn't push into your skin.
- Make sure the tape measure is level all the way around.
- Relax, exhale, and measure your waist, but don't suck in your stomach.

If your waist measures 35 inches or more, you need to lose weight and are at risk for health problems. (Men should have a waist measurement of no more than 40 inches.) If your waist measures some-

WOMEN			
HEIGHT FEET INCHES	SMALL FRAME	MEDIUM FRAME	LARGE FRAME
4' 10"	102–111	109–121	118–131
4' 11"	103–113	111–123	120–134
5' 0"	104–115	113–126	122–137
5' 1"	106–118	115–129	125–140
5' 2"	108–121	118–132	128–143
5' 3"	111–124	121–135	131–147
5' 4"	114–127	124–138	134–151
5' 5"	117–130	127–141	137–155
5' 6"	120–133	130–144	140–159
5' 7"	123–136	133–147	143–163
5' 8"	126–139	136–150	146–167
5' 9"	129–142	139–153	149–170
5' 10"	132–145	142–156	152–173
5' 11"	135–148	145–159	155–176
6' 0"	138–151	148–162	158–179

Weights at ages 25–59 based on lowest mortality. Weight in pounds according to frame (in indoor clothing weighing 3 lbs.; shoes with 1" heels).

where between 30 and 34 inches, you can still benefit from losing weight, even if you're in the clear for health problems.

FAT HABIT #5

I'm a junk food addict. —SHELLY T.

It turns out, this isn't just exaggeration. Fast food can cause addictionlike qualities, especially among susceptible individuals. When some people eat fast food, the feel-good response that occurs in the brain triggers them to go back for more.

Research from the Scripps Research Institute in Jupiter, Florida, found that animals with unlimited access to foods similar to fast-food offerings developed addictionlike eating behaviors and binge eating, compared with animals fed a healthy diet or those with limited exposure to the junk food. The animals would binge on junk food, and they gained a significant amount of fat.

SLIM SOLUTION

LIMIT FAST FOOD

If you know that fast food is a trigger food for you, try to limit your exposure to fast-food restaurants. Although this may be challenging—you may not be able to drive more than a few miles without passing a McDonald's or a Taco Bell—it takes only a few times of doing so before your cravings subside. Just think, soon enough you'll easily be able to drive by instead of driving through! In the meantime, use these tips to help dodge the drive-through:

- *Map out alternative routes so you avoid passing the normal pit stops.* Skip those freeway exits that are essentially express lanes to fast-food outlets. And when you're at the mall or airports, steer clear of the food court areas.
- *Allow yourself an occasional fast-food meal.* Choose the number of fast-food meals that you'll allow yourself to have each week or month—that way, you're limiting your intake without depriving yourself. We recommend eating out no more than twice a week, whenever possible. Once you go a couple days without fast food, you'll start to realize it was just a habit, and you can, in fact, live without it.
- *Choose wisely.* When you do get a fast-food fix, be sure to use our advice for making the best choices (see Chapter 6 for more solutions on dining out).
- *Make your own fast food.* Whip up healthy versions of your favorite meals so you can satisfy your cravings without blowing

your calorie budget. A turkey or lean beef burger with baked sweet-potato fries is one of our favorite meals—and it really satisfies that desire for fast food.

FAT HABIT #6

I just keep losing and regaining . . . again and again. —ROBIN R.

You lose the weight—hooray, you feel fabulous. You gain it back (and maybe more!)—ugh, how depressing! It's a vicious cycle that millions of dieters are stuck in. Research shows that losing weight is the easy part—it's keeping it off that's the real work.

SLIM SOLUTIONS

AIM SMALL

Bigger isn't always better when it comes to weight loss. In fact, one of the best ways to ensure that you don't regain lost weight is to lose no more than 5 percent of your current body weight at a time. (If you weigh 150 pounds, that's 7.5 pounds.) When you maintain that weight for six months, then—and only then—should you consider trying to lose another 5 percent. Weight maintenance requires more energy and focus than weight loss, so it's important to learn how to live in your lighter body for six months before trying to lose more weight.

MOVE MORE

You gotta move it to lose it—and keep on moving to keep it off. Research shows that people who've successfully maintained their weight loss exercise sixty to ninety minutes a day. Here's why activity—and usually even more activity than you needed to peel off those pounds—is a key ingredient in weight maintenance: When you lose weight, your metabolic rate drops. Exercise counterbalances this drop. If you're not that active right now, strive for thirty to forty-five minutes a day, most days a week. The best type of exercise for helping you stay slimmer is a combination of aerobic exercise, high-intensity interval training, and strength training.

These three are a true triple threat: Aerobic exercise helps burn calories; interval training results in greater boosts to your metabolic rate compared with lower-intensity exercise; while strength training helps build muscle tissue, which burns more calories at rest than fat tissue. Muscles and the cardiovascular system adapt to exercise workloads quickly, so be sure to change up your routine frequently.

STEP ON YOUR SCALE

Another secret of successful losers: They've made peace with their bathroom scales. In fact, they step on it weekly to help prevent pounds from creeping back. (It's not necessary to weigh yourself more than once a week—doing so may only drive you crazy.) If your scale is covered in dust, brush it off and put it to good use. Remember, pounds come off slowly but are quick to pile back on, so as soon as you see the needle start heading north, do what you did to lose the weight in the first place, so you can quickly correct course.

LOG IT

Talk about the power of the pen: Keeping a diet journal—either on paper or online—helps you stay on track. Jotting down your meals and snacks will help you identify what you're doing right and wrong. For instance, one of the major reasons people regain lost weight is that they revert back to their old diet. There's no denying it when it's right there in black-and-white: You see "brownies" and "beer" instead of the healthier "berries" and "beans" that used to make up your diet.

CUT BACK ON DINING OUT AND DRINKING

Every meal eaten out ups your odds of gaining back those lost pounds. Successful dieters tend to take control over what they eat, preparing most of their meals and snacks at home. If you limited meals out and alcohol while you lost weight, you can't expect to maintain that loss by frequenting restaurants and enjoying cocktails more than a few times a week.

EAT A PROTEIN-PACKED BREAKFAST

Thinking about downing a giant Danish for breakfast, or worse, skipping the meal altogether? Forget about it! One of the most consistent strategies for maintaining a leaner frame is eating a protein-rich breakfast. In fact, some studies suggest that replacing poor-quality carbohydrates with lean protein can help shift your metabolism and hunger hormones, making your goal weight easier to maintain. At the very least, start your day right with a protein-packed meal that contains limited sweets. Use our favorite hunger-curbing breakfasts found in Chapter 7. We make sure that our recommended breakfasts contain at least 20 grams of protein, or nearly 25 percent of the meal's calories, so you feel fuller, longer.

For more solutions to keep the weight off, see Fat Habit #29, "I'm a yo-yo dieter."

FAT HABIT #7

I have to take medications that cause me to gain weight. —ALYSSA T.

It's true: Some diseases and conditions as well as certain medications are associated with weight gain. However, that doesn't mean that we don't have a Slim Solution for this issue.

Several types of drug have the unwanted side effect of weight gain. This includes certain types of antidepressants, diabetes drugs, blood pressure pills, and steroids, among others.

Does this mean you're destined to be heavy as long as you're under doctor's orders? Absolutely not! Use the strategies below to stay on track.

SLIM SOLUTIONS

CHECK THE LABEL

You can find detailed information—including (both potential and probable) side effects like weight loss—for prescription meds. If you don't see "weight changes" or "weight gain" listed on the label, ask the pharmacist whether weight gain is associated with your medication.

CHECK IN WITH YOUR MD

If you know or suspect that you've gained weight due to a medication, speak with your health care provider. At the very least, he can change dosages, timing, or combinations of medicines to help. In other cases, he may be able to prescribe a comparable alternative. For example, metformin is a popular diabetes drug that is not associated with weight gain; and for depression, Wellbutrin, Zyban, and Serzone don't seem to cause weight gain.

If you're stuck taking a medication that's associated with weight gain, you have a few ways to help prevent pound rebound. For starters, eating a healthy diet (as outlined in Chapter 4) can not only improve your condition, but it may also help reduce the amount of some medications you take. Small changes in body weight (just 5 percent of your current weight) are achievable for most people— even those on medications linked with weight gain. Finally, focus on the long-term health benefits you can gain from eating well, rather than what you see on the scale. Highlight how you feel, how

---

Pills That May Pack on the Pounds

Antidepressants
Elavil, Luvox, Paxil, Prozac, Remeron, Sarafem, Surmontil, Tofranil, Vanatrip, Zoloft, Zyprexa

Antihistamines
Benadryl, Nytol

Antiseizure/Antipsychotic
Clozaril, Depakote, Haldol, Loxitane, Risperdal, Zyprexa

Diabetes
DiaBeta, Diabinese

Heart Disease
Cardura, Inderal, Lopressor, Minipress, Tenormin

Steroids
Prednisone

---

much energy you have, how much better your condition is, or what you are able to accomplish physically, rather than highlighting your body weight.

FAT HABIT #8

I have depression, and the thought of trying to eat right and exercise is just too overwhelming. —TARA R.

Obesity and depression often go hand in hand—but there has been a sort of chicken-and-egg debate about which comes first. Many people assume that being fat is depressing, especially in our culture, where thin is in. However, based on some early research, it seems that being depressed may cause you to gain weight. A study published in the *American Journal of Public Health* found that people who reported symptoms of depression, like feeling sad or hopeless, gained weight more rapidly over a fifteen-year period and accrued more belly fat than those who appeared to be happier. While it is not fully understood why depression may be causing weight gain, there are several theories. When you're depressed, you tend to be inactive and, in some cases, eat more. Some antidepressant medications may also cause weight gain. It's also possible that the stress hormone cortisol, which promotes fat storage, may be more active in depressed people. This is pretty disheartening news, considering that one in every ten Americans suffers from depression, according to the Centers for Disease Control and Prevention.

Regardless of which one comes first, there's no doubt depression can interfere with weight loss and maintenance. Plus, you might feel like you do not have the physical or emotional strength to get motivated.

SLIM SOLUTION

GET HELP

The first step toward recovery is to *seek professional help*. Depression is a medical illness that is best treated using a multifaceted approach that consists of talk therapy, exercise, stress reduction and meditative techniques, and medications.

Taking care of your mental well-being will enable you to focus on lifestyle changes in eating, activity, and stress management, which can help you shed pounds. Don't get discouraged if therapy doesn't seem to work right away—treatment takes time.

FAT HABIT #9

I can't live *without my diet soda.* —PHIL G.

A sweet treat that provides no calories? Sign us up! That's the allure of diet soda (and any other product made with artificial sweeteners). And we're gulping down plenty of it—an average of 27 ounces a day, or slightly more than two cans, according to research. We're also gobbling up more artificial sweeteners in cookies, yogurt, and other products.

Not coincidentally, rates of obesity have risen. That may be because many people (including Julie, in a not-too-distant life) say they become addicted to artificially sweetened products—they feel like they *need* it every day. Experts believe diet soda and other diet products are "addictive" because they sometimes contain caffeine (which can be addicting) and provide a supersweet taste. Another factor: our beliefs and behaviors. For instance, some people view diet beverages as a reward—"I deserve a diet soda for working out"—while others reason, "It's a not-so-bad habit, relatively speaking. Instead of a cigarette, I'll just drink a glass of diet soda."

If it doesn't contain any calories, then what's the harm? The constant intense sweetness of diet sodas and other treats that contain sugar substitutes makes it harder for us to enjoy the natural sweetness found in an apple, orange, sweet potato, or corn. Not to mention these supersweet sweeteners fuel your desire for more and more intensely sweet treats.

Plus, slurping down a soda that contains artificial sweeteners instead of a caloric sugary beverage may help lower calorie intake, but there's no evidence that it helps you keep off the pounds in the long term, reports a recent review of hundreds of studies on noncaloric sweeteners, appetite, and food intake published in the *American*

Journal of Clinical Nutrition. In fact, two recent studies found that being a diet soda drinker can make you heavier. Those who drank three servings or more of diet soda a day—at least twenty-one weekly servings—were almost twice as likely to become overweight or obese after seven to eight years as people who skipped sipping diet drinks, according to researchers at the University of Texas Health Science Center in San Antonio. And people who consumed at least one daily serving of diet soda (versus none) were more likely to develop a high waist circumference, which is linked with type 2 diabetes, hypertension, and cardiovascular disease, according to a recent study.

Researchers are debating whether there's an actual psychological and/or physical addiction with diet soda. If you've ever craved one and/or experienced withdrawal symptoms when you try to steer clear, you probably don't need scientific proof. How to break your addiction? Read on for some helpful hints.

SLIM SOLUTIONS

CUT BACK

If you suffer from a diet soda dependence, we believe that cutting back to no more than 12 ounces a day is a good idea.

CHOOSE YOUR QUIT METHOD

There are two approaches to breaking your diet soda addiction: Quit cold turkey or wean yourself off. Both work and are completely valid. To quit cold turkey, refer to Fat Habit #3, "I'm addicted to all things sweet." If you want to gradually wean yourself off of diet sodas, start by setting a limit, like 12 ounces total per day, and then plan for and enjoy it. When you feel like you can go several days without getting a fizzy fix, then you've essentially beat your "addiction." As long as you're struggling to lose or maintain a healthy weight, keep your use of diet beverages to a minimum.

I'm nearly 50 years old . . . if I even smell fatty foods
now, I'll gain weight. —SOPHIE T.

We'd like to let you in on a little secret: We're *all* getting older, and there's nothing anyone can do about it. While you have to accept the fact that you can't outrun Father Time, you don't have to accept weight gain as part of the aging process.

Preventing middle-age spread will not only keep you from jumping up a size or two; it can also protect your health. Weight gain during middle age has been linked to diabetes, heart disease, and even some cancers. In one large study, middle-aged women and men who gained 11 to 22 pounds after age 20 were up to three times more likely to develop heart disease, high blood pressure, type 2 diabetes, and gallstones than those who gained 5 pounds or fewer. Those who gained more than 22 pounds had an even larger risk of developing these diseases.

Sure, your metabolic rate slows over time (you'll burn about 100 fewer calories per day at age 40 than you did at age 25), but there are many other contributors to midlife weight gain, including life. As we age, our lives become more complicated, whether it's with children, work, or aging parents. Simply put, being a full-fledged adult leaves less time for focusing on fitness and healthy eating.

SLIM SOLUTIONS

SET ASIDE SOME "ME" TIME

There are two ways to combat weight gain as we get older: Exercise more and/or eat less. Research shows that older Americans who exercise the most are least likely to gain weight over time. Your goal: 60 minutes a day to maintain or lose weight. And keep in mind that declines in metabolism are nothing compared with the number of

40 Ways to Cut 100 Calories

AT BREAKFAST

- Eat breakfast. Those who start with a morning meal eat fewer calories over the course of the day.
- Reduce (by half) the amount of sweetener you use in your coffee, tea, or cereal.
- Use a nonstick skillet and cooking spray in place of butter or margarine to prepare your eggs.
- Spread your muffin, bagel, or toast with 2 tablespoons of fat-free cream cheese in place of regular cream cheese.
- Substitute no-sugar-added jelly or jam for the sugar-rich varieties.
- Select lean ham, turkey, or Canadian bacon instead of regular sausage or pork bacon.
- Fill your omelet with onions, peppers, spinach, and mushrooms instead of cheese and meat.
- Lighten up your omelet, frittata, or scrambled eggs by using 4 egg whites or ½ cup of egg substitute.
- Order a smaller-size coffee drink.

AT LUNCH AND DINNER

- Start your meal with a piece of fruit or a tossed salad.
- Make your sandwich with light, whole-wheat bread.
- Add fresh zucchini, green peppers, mushrooms, and onions to spaghetti sauce instead of meat.
- Put lettuce, tomato, onions, and pickles on your burger or sandwich instead of cheese.
- Prepare tuna or chicken salad with fat-free mayonnaise.
- Grill your sandwich using nonstick cooking spray or reduced-calorie trans fat–free margarine in place of butter.
- Stuff a pita pocket with more fresh vegetables, less meat and cheese.
- Opt for water-packed tuna instead of tuna packed in oil.
- Select a portion-controlled frozen entrée in place of a burger and fries.

- Trade regular butter for a light whipped or low-calorie butter substitute.
- Make a pizza with half the cheese.
- Select soft taco–size (6- to 8-inch) flour tortillas instead of the larger burrito size.
- Substitute fat-free sour cream in recipes.
- Choose 1 percent cottage cheese in place of regular.
- Skim the fat off soups, stews, and sauces before serving.
- Leave three to four bites on your plate.
- Go for thin-crust over thick-crust pizza.
- Downsize your plates or bowls.
- Enjoy an open-faced sandwich topped with leaf lettuce instead of bread.
- Have 2 ounces of baked tortilla chips with salsa instead of fried, full-fat chips.

AT DESSERT

- Satisfy your sweet tooth with a sliver, bite, or taste of dessert instead of a full portion.
- Make your own root-beer float with sugar-free root beer and light ice cream.
- Freeze blended fresh fruit into a sorbet for a refreshing dessert.
- Leave the cone at the counter; have a single-dip ice-cream scoop in a cup.
- Choose your piece of sheet cake from the middle, where there's less icing.
- Top angel food cake with berries instead of icing or chocolate sauce.
- Cut your slice of cake or pie in half.
- Dish up reduced-calorie ice cream or frozen yogurt in place of regular ice cream.
- Enjoy a dish of fresh fruit that's in season instead of custard or pudding.
- Have a cup of fresh grapes instead of ½ cup of raisins.
- Have a virgin drink instead of an alcoholic one.

calories in food, so simply monitoring what, when, how much, and why you're eating—and cutting back—can easily accommodate minor metabolic dips.

CUT 100 CALORIES AFTER 40

To maintain your weight after age 40, you're going to have to eat 100 fewer calories per day. Let's be honest: 100 calories isn't all that much. Plus, with a few creative switches and swaps (see sidebar on the previous pages), you can eliminate these calories without missing a thing.

PUMP IT UP

Turn your body into a calorie-burning machine by increasing your muscle mass. As we mentioned earlier, adding just five pounds of muscle can help you burn 50 more calories a day. Aim for at least forty to sixty minutes of strength training twice per week. Use the weight room at your local gym, or exercise with dumbbells, resistance bands, or even your own body weight at home. Never strength-trained before? Sign up for a few sessions with a personal trainer; he or she can help you learn how to perform—and get the most out of—each move, as well as avoid injury. Once you've been at it for a while, you'll need to increase the weight or resistance you're using.

FILL UP IN THE A.M.

Breakfast skimpers ("Just coffee and dry toast, please") and skippers are making a major metabolic mistake: eating too little to flip on their metabolism switch, as well as the "satisfaction switch" in the brain that registers fullness in the stomach.

If you typically bypass breakfast, it may be because you overate

Got 10 Minutes? That's Enough for a Healthy Breakfast!

- **Oatmeal yum.** Top 1 cup plain oatmeal with 2 tablespoons each of chopped nuts and dried fruit, a pinch of cinnamon, and a drizzle of honey.
- **"Egg-lish" muffin crostini and cheese.** Put 1 poached egg, 1 slice of lean ham, and 1 thin (½ ounce) slice of Swiss cheese on ½ toasted whole-wheat English muffin.
- **B & B bruschetta.** Top 1 slice of whole-wheat toast with 1 tablespoon of all-natural nut butter, ½ sliced banana, and a drizzle of honey.
- **Cereal and fruit.** Pour 1 cup skim milk (or calcium-fortified soy milk) over 1 cup high-fiber, whole-grain cereal and serve with ½ pink or red grapefruit on the side.
- **Waffle wise.** Toast 2 low-fat whole-grain frozen waffles with ½ cup of fresh (or thawed, unsweetened frozen) berries and 1 tablespoon of maple syrup.
- **"Egg-lish" muffin and greens.** Stuff 1 whole-wheat English muffin with 1 cooked egg, 1 slice cooked Canadian bacon, watercress or baby spinach, and a squirt of lemon.
- **Cheese toast.** Top a slice of whole-wheat toast with 1 slice part-skim mozzarella cheese with a few fresh basil leaves; serve with 1 cup low-sodium 100 percent vegetable juice (add a few drops of hot sauce for eye-opening pizzazz).
- **Berry smoothie.** Blend 1 cup low-fat Greek yogurt, ½ cup berries, ½ cup 100 percent apple juice, and ½ cup crushed ice until smooth.
- **Greek yogurt and jam.** Mix ½ cup low-fat Greek yogurt with 1 tablespoon 100 percent fruit spread or jam of your choice.
- **Energy pita.** Top ½ whole-grain pita with Neufchâtel (light cream) cheese, 2 tablespoons chopped nuts, and 2 tablespoons dried fruit.

the night before and just aren't hungry, or you're trying to cut calories by missing a meal. But research shows you might want to rethink your approach. It's worth cutting off nighttime eating and saving those calories for your morning meal. When researchers at the University of Texas at El Paso analyzed the food diaries of 867 women and men, they found that study volunteers who had a bigger meal in the morning went on to eat 100 to 200 fewer calories later in the day. Research from Michigan State University that tracked 4,218 people showed that women who skipped breakfast were 30 percent more likely to be overweight.

Let's put it this way: No one has gotten fat from eating a healthy breakfast—but many have become thin. Research shows that some 78 percent of successful dieters almost always eat breakfast, compared with just 4 percent who rarely eat it. "Front-loading" your calories is one of the easiest ways to lose weight.

Aim to have breakfast within two hours of waking up, and choose one that contains protein and fiber, says Patricia Bannan, MS, RD, author of *Eat Right When Time Is Tight: 150 Slim-Down Strategies and No-Cook Food Fixes*. Check out the sidebar on the previous page for some of Bannan's favorite no-fuss breakfasts.

STRESS LESS

Before you file this away in the easier-said-than-done folder, realize that stress can significantly undermine your healthy eating and exercise habits. When things get hectic, your levels of the stress hormone cortisol shoot up, which can trigger cravings for high-fat, high-carb foods. The worst part: Your body sends extra fat to your waistline. Millions of years ago, when food was scarce and marauding bears were plentiful, this metabolic trick came in pretty handy— it protected you from threats and gave you the energy to scavenge for sustenance. But in this era of chronic stress (job, kids, house, spouse) and twenty-four/seven access to all-you-can-eat food, that extra cortisol could easily lead to mammoth overeating. To help get your stress in check, read the sidebar below.

Tension-Taming Tips from RDs

How do nutrition pros handle stress? A good yoga class is how Katherine unwinds, and Julie likes to sweat out her anxieties at CrossFit. Check out how a few other busy RDs chill out when things get crazy:

"Who said you need quiet to relax? I love to pop in a favorite CD and dance for a few songs. It leaves me feeling ready to take on the world. I also love a cup of coffee around nine-thirty a.m., after the kids are off to school and before I get to work." —Ilaria St. Florian, MS, RD

"I 'write it all out.' Every night I jot down happenings, thoughts, and things accomplished that day, including my frustrations. I find that when my mind is 'cleaned up,' it is easier to relax and fall asleep." —Chris Cooper, MS, RD

"After my kids go to bed, I usually take a bubble bath and read a fitness or food magazine and soak up the suds." —Kitty Broihier, MS, RD

■

FAT HABIT #11

I've hit menopause—it's useless to try to diet. —TINA C.

Menopause and the years leading up to it (known as perimenopause) are a serious dieting danger zone. If you don't step up your exercise and watch what you eat, you'll likely gain a pound per year during this time—and much of the fat will wind up in your waist.

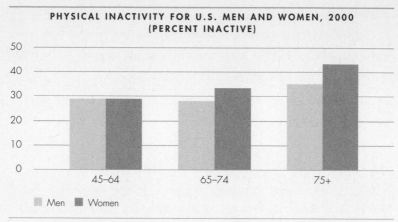

PHYSICAL INACTIVITY FOR U.S. MEN AND WOMEN, 2000 (PERCENT INACTIVE)

Men   Women

Source: Behavioral Risk Factor Surveillance Survey. Centers for Disease Control and Prevention, National Center for Chronic Disease Prevention and Health Promotion. www.cdc.gov/brfss/

The "menopause middle," as it's lovingly called, is a result of the normal fat distribution pattern that occurs when the production of sex hormones declines. As you probably know, belly fat is a real health risk. Excess weight in your abdomen boosts your risk for heart disease and certain cancers.

But there's some good news: Abdominal fat is more readily used as fuel than fat that's stored in other areas of the body. Besides, you don't have to accept the menopause middle as your weight fate. Think of it this way: By the time menopause rolls around, women often have fewer demands on their time than when they were in their twenties and thirties. You may also be more settled in your career and have more flexibility with your work life. Take advantage of this downtime by finding fun and creative ways to exercise. Studies have found that even more than hormones and age, a *sedentary lifestyle* is the biggest culprit in postmenopause weight gain. People tend to decrease their level of physical activity as they get older.

As the chart on the previous page indicates, few older adults get the minimum recommended thirty or more minutes of moderate physical activity five or more days per week. Nearly 30 percent of adults aged 45 to 64 are inactive, meaning they engage in no leisure-time physical activity. Women were more likely than men to report no leisure-time activity.

SLIM SOLUTIONS

GET ACTIVE

Simply put, women who maintain or increase physical activity prior to, during, and after menopause are going to gain less weight. Now is the time to take up that sport you always wanted to try: Join a tennis league or a swim group, or even train for your first marathon!

DON'T FORGET DIET

It is important to remember that it's the combination of both diet and exercise that will keep you trim throughout menopause and beyond. The Women's Healthy Lifestyle Project, a five-year study that followed women through menopause, concluded that women who ate a low-calorie diet *and* got regular exercise lost weight, while women who did not watch their diet or exercise gained an average of 5 pounds after one year.

The women in the diet and exercise group ate about 1,300 calories a day and dedicated themselves to regular moderate-intensity exercise, such as walking briskly 10 to 15 miles a week. In contrast, surveys show that American women are eating just under 1,900 calories a day. And we've already covered just how little exercise they're getting—nearly one in three women over age 45 is physically inactive.

FAT HABIT #12

I'm just big-boned. —AMY W.

"Big-boned" is a bit like "curvy"—both can be used to accurately describe a woman's build, or they can be used as an excuse for carrying around a few extra pounds.

Is everyone in your family big and tall? If so, it might be completely fine for you to weigh more, because you may have more lean body mass (bone and muscle) compared with someone with a slight frame. If, on the other hand, you're using this term to cover up the fact that you have some excess body fat, then you may have a real problem.

SLIM SOLUTIONS

FIND YOUR FRAME

Determine whether you are, indeed, big-boned. View Fat Habit #4, "I'm a curvy woman," to figure out your frame. If you simply have a bigger frame, you may have to settle on a slightly higher weight than you may like. Instead of obsessing, use other measures (see below for some examples) to gauge your progress.

KNOW YOUR NUMBERS

If you are big-boned, it's best to use a combination of scale weight and other measures, including BMI and body fat, to determine how healthy you are. How do you find out these numbers? BMI requires using a simple formula, given below; you have a few options for body fat.

BMI CALCULATOR

Figuring out your BMI involves a simple calculation using your height and weight (www.cdc.gov/healthyweight/assessing/bmi/index.html).

Simply plug these two numbers into a BMI calculator to learn whether you are obese, overweight, or normal weight.

Note: The BMI was developed using large, population-based studies. Though it doesn't address percentage of body fat or muscle, it helps health care professionals quickly assess which patients may be at risk for health problems linked to excess weight.

Pros: Free and readily available; good for assessing health risks.

Cons: Doesn't measure body-fat percentage; if you are short or very muscular, results tend to be less accurate.

BODY FAT–MEASURING SCALES

Bioelectrical impedance analysis technology has been added to traditional bathroom scales. The scales send a harmless electrical current up through your body to "read" the amount of fat body mass and lean body mass, calculating your percentage of body fat.

Pros: Moderate in price at $50 to $200 per scale; convenient.

Cons: Bioelectrical impedance scales are sensitive to the amount of fluids in your body—even your menstrual cycle may affect the reading. It's important to strictly follow the guidelines for weighing yourself, including time of day, and fluid and food intake. Most home bioelectrical impedance scales are not highly accurate.

DEXA SCANNING

DEXA stands for "dual-energy X-ray absorptiometry," the same imaging technology doctors use to measure bone density and determine osteoporosis risk. During the test, you lie on an X-ray table for about ten minutes while the scanner measures your body fat, muscle, and bone mineral density.

Pros: Noninvasive; one of the most accurate measures of body fat available. DEXA also shows the location of fat deposits in specific body regions, which is important because *where* your body stores fat can be much more indicative of disease risk than *how much* fat you carry.

Cons: DEXA tests are expensive (they can range from $200 to more than $500), and most health insurance policies will not pay for this test as a way to measure body fat. DEXA is usually available only through a physician.

UNDERWATER TESTING

Underwater testing, also known as hydrodensitometry testing, involves getting into a tank filled with water. Based on the amount of water you displace, your body density and body fat can be calculated.

Pros: This test is considered the gold standard of body fat measurement.

Cons: It can be inconvenient to find an underwater testing unit (many are located at universities).

BOD POD

The BOD POD is a relatively new tool that relies on air displacement to determine body fat. There's no submersion (you don't get wet)—you simply step into a chamber.

Pros: Relatively inexpensive at $45 to $65 per test; more convenient than underwater weighing. Under the right conditions, you can achieve accuracy within a few percentage points.

Cons: Hydration and other factors can affect test results; not as accurate as underwater testing or DEXA.

THE TAPE MEASURE

It's one of the oldest obesity tests, because it's a basic indicator of body fat. It's important to measure at your belly button, not at the thinnest point of your waist, and to measure on the exhale. Men with measurements higher than 40 centimeters, or women with waist measurements higher than 35 centimeters, are considered at risk for a variety of diseases.

Pros: It's free, easy, and serves as a decent measure for assessing risk for chronic diseases like diabetes, heart disease, and stroke.

Cons: It won't give you your exact body fat percentage (it simply indicates whether you're carrying extra weight around your middle).

SKIN-FOLD CALIPERS

Most health clubs offer this test; it's the most widely used method for measuring body fat. Essentially it's a "pinch" test using a measuring device at several points on the body, like the thighs, hips, and upper arm.

Pros: If done properly, the skin-fold test can be reasonably accurate. Most health clubs will do this test for free or for a small fee.

Cons: Accuracy depends on the skill of the person conducting the test; if the tester is inexperienced, your reading may be way off.

HEIGHT/WEIGHT CHARTS

These are the simple height-versus-weight tables used for years by many insurance companies.

Pros: They are easy to find and you can use them on your own.

Cons: They are not necessarily the best indicator of health risks.

FAT HABIT #13

I'm always hungry. —MISSY C.

It's biologically impossible to lose weight without feeling some amount of hunger. It all comes down to hunger management—how well you do it can determine how successful you are at losing weight and keeping it off.

SLIM SOLUTIONS

DETERMINE THE CAUSE OF YOUR HUNGER

Some people who are always "hungry" may be mistaking food for love or support; if you're unable to find the love and support you need through your relationships, you may feel hungry or unsatisfied and turn to food for comfort. In some cases, a diet that is rich in junk foods or treats triggers intense cravings and makes it almost impossible to manage your hunger. Another common cause: skipping meals. If you miss meals or don't eat regularly (every three to four hours), hunger could rear its ugly head.

USE THE HUNGER SCALE

All of us have the innate ability to control calories—you just have to listen to your body. To get back in touch with your body's hunger and fullness signals, you can try using the hunger scale, as shown on the following page.

How can the hunger scale help? Your body metabolizes and uses foods best when you eat the right amounts at the right times. In addition to helping you cut calories, the scale can also help you curb cravings. You can also say buh-bye to binge foods—the scale will help you eat only when you're physically hungry. Most binges, on the other hand, stem from emotional reasons.

How does it work? Try to eat when your body feels like a 4 on

THE HUNGER SCALE

1.	You're so hungry you'll eat anything.
2.	You can't ignore your hunger and everything looks and sounds good to eat.
3.	Your stomach is growling and you have hunger pangs.
4.	**You can feel you're getting hungry and it's time to think about what to eat.**
5.	**You're neither hungry nor full.**
6.	**Just right; you're satisfied but could easily eat more.**
7.	**Totally satisfied; hunger is gone and you won't be hungry for hours.**
8.	You're full and don't want anything else to eat.
9.	You feel stuffed and uncomfortable.
10.	You're painfully full and may even feel sick.

©2013 Appetite for Health (appforHealth.com)

 Assess your hunger and fullness before, during, and after your meals and snacks. Try to stay within the shaded areas (numbers 4–7) to help keep portions and calories in check.

the scale and stop when it's about 6 or 7. You want to avoid being so hungry (a 3 or lower) that you overeat, and at the same time, you don't want to chow down until you feel ready-to-unzip-my-pants full (8 or higher).

Keep a food journal for five to seven days, and make sure you note where your hunger is, from 1 to 10, before and after eating. Try to keep your hunger controlled and within the 4-to-7 range on the scale. (When you wake up, it's okay if you're a 2.)

When you're eating, take a few minutes to pause during the meal to assess your hunger. If you're still below a 6, continue eating. Remember, it takes fifteen to twenty minutes for the stomach to provide the brain signals of fullness, so don't speed-eat! Get to know your body and when you need to stop eating to reach the feeling of 7 after a meal.

After a week, you should start to develop a healthier relationship with food and be more attuned to listening for—and feeding—your hunger. Use the scale for as long as you think you need it.

FAT HABIT #14

My whole family is this way. —STACIE L.

If you're like most Americans, one or both of your parents are plump. As it turns out, the apple doesn't fall too far from the not-so-trim tree: When one or both parents are overweight, you're more likely to be overweight too. In fact, girls who have two overweight parents have been shown to be eight times more likely to be overweight by age 13.

It's a question of nature versus nurture: Is it genes that predispose these kids to obesity, or is it their environment that makes them pack on pounds? Researchers have found that it has more to do with the food environment than genetic makeup. Parents who are overweight may teach young children unhealthy food habits—like eating when they're not hungry, eating to avoid problems or emotional issues, using "food as love," serving Costco-size portions, and cooking less frequently—compared with households with parents who are at a healthier weight.

The problem is that most parents don't even realize they're setting their kids up for weight failure. Surprisingly, most parents don't even realize when their kids *are* overweight. A recent poll found that while the majority of Americans believe that childhood obesity is a "significant and growing challenge for the country," a whopping 84 percent say their children are at a healthy weight—despite national stats showing that nearly one-third of children and teens are overweight or obese.

SLIM SOLUTIONS

EVALUATE YOUR EATING HABITS

It's all too easy to blame your family for your weight woes. Sure, genes play a role, but in many cases, the eating habits you've learned from an early age are the real culprit. Keep a food log to determine how and when you eat. Do you consume a lot more food when you're stressed? Do you eat when you're happy? A food log can help pinpoint your problems with food.

START YOUR OWN HEALTHY HABITS

You—and you alone—are responsible for what you eat, your weight, and the life you live. No matter how dysfunctional the food environment you grew up in was, start to create your own healthy habits and traditions. Your first step: using the resources throughout this book.

IT'S *THEIR* FAULT!

WE'D BE THE LAST PEOPLE TO URGE YOU TO PASS THE BUCK— BUT IF you've been struggling to slim down, it's important to take a look around you at the company you've been keeping.

All excuses aside, the people you are in the habit of spending time with, including your significant other, family, friends, colleagues, your boss, even your online friends and social media, could be sabotaging your diet. Recent research reveals that weight gain can be "socially contagious," so we'll need you to take a good look at who is influencing your day-to-day choices, and we'll help you find Slim Solutions that will help you outsmart the savviest diet saboteurs in your life.

FAT HABIT #15

Doesn't anyone listen to me when I say, "I'm on a diet!"?
Sheesh, why don't they get it? —MARYBETH T.

Does it seem like everyone is conspiring against you? It's almost as if they don't want you to lose weight. "They" includes: Your mom, who asks, "Don't you want a piece of chocolate cake? I stayed up all night making it for you." Your work colleague, who thinks he's being helpful when he announces, "We left a plate of sandwiches and cookies in the kitchen. Go help yourself." Your pal, who pleads, "Have another drink with me—I don't want to drink alone." Even your spouse, who tries to negotiate, "Forget the fish. Let's have steak for dinner tonight."

It's hard enough to withstand the many temptations you're faced with day in and day out without having to also face down a squad of diet saboteurs. How to keep your diet and relationships intact? Use the advice below, and who knows—you may even influence them to break a few bad habits of their own in the process.

SLIM SOLUTIONS

BREAK THE NEWS

Simply tell friends and family that you're trying to improve your diet and health. Explain that you hope they will respect your decision and that they will do their best to support you on your journey. This offers a two-for-one benefit: Not only does it make them aware of how they influence your eating and exercise habits, but it also makes you more accountable for your actions. Another perk: You have a built-in support system to turn to when times get tough. Several studies show that dieters who enlist the support of others are more successful at losing weight and keeping it off. It's one of the reasons why the major weight-loss programs (like Weight Watchers and Jenny Craig) require in-person or online check-ins.

BE SPECIFIC ABOUT HOW THEY CAN SUPPORT YOU

Need a cheerleader in your corner? Prefer to have a drill sergeant on your side? Tell your friends and family how they can go about helping you. If you could use a gentle nudge whenever you slack off—say, skipping a workout—ask them to be firm but encouraging with you. If, on the other hand, you'd rather not have their feedback, just ask them to hold their tongues. You can say, "I'd rather you not pass comments when I have a piece of candy or a handful of chips. I've allowed myself some treat calories every day and have been doing pretty well so far."

MAKE ALTERNATIVE PLANS

Pinpoint your potential pitfalls and come up with alternate plans. If you normally have coffee and pastries with a pal each week, tell her you'd rather connect over a walk instead. If work lunches with coworkers end up costing you more calories than you'd care to spend, ask your colleagues whether you can bring your own lunch and eat in the office cafeteria together. This way you're removing the opportunity for them to undermine your efforts.

SWAP ADVICE

Having a support network means you have others with whom you can share your experiences—both good and bad. People who check in with a dietitian or other health care professional experience better weight-loss results. Even online check-ins result in more pounds lost, so using virtual resources from commercial weight-loss programs or sites like SparkPeople, Lose It!, or MyFitnessPal can help you reach your goals and provide much-needed support.

Diet BFFs Double Weight Loss or Team Up to Slim Down

The old cliché "There's strength in numbers" is certainly true when it comes to weight loss. One study from Brown University found that dieters with diet buddies lost significantly more weight at six, twelve, and eighteen months compared with those who tried to slim down solo.

How to pick a pal? Opt for quality over quantity. It's more important to have one buddy who's really committed than to have a handful who are only partly invested in achieving their goals and helping you achieve yours, the researchers found.

To find a diet buddy who will improve your odds of success, look for someone who you know has a can-do winning attitude that you admire. Explain to her what you're trying to do and assess whether she'd be up for the challenge too. Diet BFFs can be found pretty much anywhere: someone among your group of friends, someone in an exercise class, a neighbor, or a work colleague.

FAT HABIT #16

I've got three kids, all under age 5, and my diet seems to be somewhere between a dirty diaper and nowhere. —KATIE P.

Mac 'n' cheese, hot dogs, pizza, chicken nuggets . . . it's standard kids' food—but just because you have kids doesn't mean you need to eat like one.

We know that moms face a number of obstacles to healthy eating. When you're caring for others, you don't have as much time for yourself. The result: You grab whatever is easiest and quickest—you know, foods like Teddy Grahams, Goldfish, and Tater Tots—or

Support SOS: Three Ways to Seek and Gain the Support to Win

"SELL" IT TO THEM

Try to encourage your friends and family to join your efforts without judging, blaming, or nagging. Position it as a chance to create something great together (a healthier self and relationship—double bonus!), and come up with rewards for yourself for every positive behavior change (a massage for a tough workout or new clothes after you've lost some weight).

GO VIRTUAL

There are many online weight-loss communities that feature message boards where people share their weight-loss tips, accomplishments, and setbacks. Ones we like: SparkPeople, Lose It!, and MyFitnessPal.

TRY SOMETHING DIFFERENT

You can't expect your weight to change if you do the same thing with the same people every day. If you need a stronger social network, visit places where you're sure to find like-minded, health-conscious individuals. Having moved numerous times as an adult, Julie has found a great network of healthy, fit friends through local running, cycling, or swimming clubs, or CrossFit gyms.

you eat whatever's left on their plate. Don't be fooled: Those kiddie calories quickly add up.

How quickly? One study found that moms ate 368 more calories per day (for a total of 2,360 calories per day) than women without children (who consumed 1,992 calories per day). Over the course of a year, that equals the calories of 38 pounds of fat! The moms also consumed more saturated fat and sugary beverages than the women without children. Dads aren't off the hook either. Another study that evaluated the diets of more than seven thousand couples found that parents ate more fat, sugar, and bread (which is often a source of empty calories) and less produce than their child-free counterparts. (In fact, the childless adults ate 5 more pounds of produce every two weeks than parents did!)

SLIM SOLUTION

Instead of feeling like your diet is doomed when you bring Junior home, let him inspire you to become a healthier eater. Once you're a parent, you become a role model for your kids, and this fact can be the inspiration you need to make positive changes in your diet. Don't believe us? Take it from a handful of RD (registered dietitian) moms, who weighed in with their best advice for feeding their kids (and themselves!) healthfully.

- *Never eat off your child's plate.* "Remember, a nibble here and a bite there add up to a lot of calories, so pay attention to what and when you are eating. If you are truly hungry, make yourself your own bowl or plate," says Stephanie Mull, MS, RD, CSSD (www.smullnutrition.net). "Also, make sure that you eat every three to four hours. Keep snacks in your car, diaper bag, and/or purse. That reduces the temptation to grab a candy bar or other high-fat, high-sugar food in the checkout line at Target because you're starving."

- *Avoid "kiddie" foods.* "Sure, kiddie foods are convenient, but most snack foods marketed to children are high in calories, sugar, or fat (or all three!), and they lack fiber and protein that help keep you satisfied," says Ruth Carey, RD, CSSD (www.ruthcarey.com). "The bottom line? Neither you nor your kids need any 'kid' foods. They can enjoy all the same healthy snack foods *you* eat, including low-fat cheese, whole-grain crackers, fruits, and vegetables."

- *Take "me" time.* "Women who make sure their own needs are being met are most successful at weight loss and are also better able to meet the needs of others," says Anne M. Fletcher, MS, RD, LD, author of the *Thin for Life* books (www.annemfletcher .com). "On the other hand, those who never take care of themselves feel resentful and wind up 'rewarding' themselves with food. Be sure to take time for things that are important for and to you."

- *Skip sweatpants.* "It's easy to ignore a gradual weight increase when your pants are expandable. Noticing how clothing fits— or, more accurately, doesn't—can help spur you to take action before it spirals out of control," says Kay Bush, RD, CD. "Busy moms may not think they can take the time to shower, dress, put on makeup, and so on, but wearing 'real' clothes kept me from packing on the pounds and just made me feel better!"

- *Play with your kids.* "When I became a mom, I did not always make it to the gym or even have a dedicated exercise routine, but what I did do every step of the way was to play along with them," says Pam Woythal, RD. "When they were toddlers, I got on scooter cars and tricycles and rode up and down the driveway with them. In the pool, we had all sorts of races, like hopping on one foot or running backward. Hey, I learned to ski at forty-two because I was taking my kids to their ski lessons every Friday and didn't want to sit in a lodge!"

- *Squeeze in fitness.* Can't get a full sweat session in? No sweat! Learn how to squeeze in short bouts of exercise. A twenty-minute walk during your lunch break, a twenty-minute march around the soccer field during your daughter's practice, and a twenty-minute stroll with the dog after dinner adds up to a solid sixty minutes of exercise, and often feels much more manageable than an hour-long gym workout. Even if you can find time only to take two fifteen-minute walks every day, you'll burn about 200 extra calories per day, or 1,400 per week, says Juliet Mancino, MS, RD, CDE, LDN. If you're getting no exercise right now, aim for 15 minutes a day. High-intensity body weight training takes only about 15 minutes, can be done at home, and will keep you fit.

- *Make the extra effort.* If only wishing away your extra weight worked. What does work for weight loss: planning ahead and putting in some effort. Make sure that each week, you've mapped out how many minutes of exercise you're going to get and have a goal for your own meals and snacks. "If you're short on sleep and haven't planned meals ahead of time, your 'exercise' and 'play' time will get gobbled up by dinner preparation and all the other unexpected chores moms need to do at the end of the day," says Suzanne Fleming, RD, LD.

- *Find what motivates you.* "I always tell my clients to find their motivation, whatever it may be, and hang on to it," says Karin Plett, RD. "Motivation makes self-discipline just a tad bit easier. My motivation is being a healthy role model for my little girl, and picturing myself at my goal weight, just knowing how good that feels."

FAT HABIT #17

*My body hasn't been the same since I gave birth to my son eighteen months ago. Now my husband and I want to try for another. —*LISA W.

Planning to have kids in the near future? Consider this: Pregnancy is one of the major risk factors for overweight and obesity, because so few women return to their prepregnancy weight. And with each subsequent pregnancy, women become pregnant at a heavier weight, creating a dangerous and hard-to-break cycle. You may have a bundle of joy on your mind, but if you're not at your ideal weight, you may want to consider postponing pregnancy for a period of time. Research shows that a woman's prepregnancy weight is even more important than how much she gains during a pregnancy when it comes to predicting postpregnancy weight.

SLIM SOLUTION

Use your desire to expand your family to help shrink your waistline. Eating a healthy diet goes beyond dropping pounds—the foods you need to eat in order to lose weight are the same foods that are important for achieving a healthy pregnancy.

To help you get to your healthy weight (see Chapter 1) before your next pregnancy, follow our meal plan guidelines (Chapter 7). And be sure to check out the advice from RD moms on how they maintain a healthy weight (Fat Habit #16, page 47).

Once you reach your ideal weight, you can think about trying for another baby. Of course, at that time you'll want to stay within the Institute of Medicine's healthy weight-gain guidelines (see chart on the next page for details). Some 43 percent of pregnant women gain more weight than the guidelines specify (37 percent gain within the range; 20 percent gain less than what's recommended). Excess weight gain is related to dangerous conditions for moms, including gestational hypertension and diabetes, as well as serious potential problems for babies, like metabolic abnormalities and low Apgar scores.

You should do whatever you can to begin your pregnancy at a healthy weight and keep your weight gain in check during your pregnancy—for you and your baby-to-be.

Optimal Pregnancy Weight Gain

Your BMI*	Recommended Weight Gain
BMI up to 19.8	28 to 40 pounds
BMI 19.8 to 26	25 to 35 pounds
BMI 26 to 29	15 to 25 pounds
BMI above 29	11 to 20 pounds
Twins	35 to 45 pounds

*See page 34.

FAT HABIT #18

I'm like a human garbage disposal—eating everything off my kids' plates after meals. —SARA B.

As tempting as it is to pop those last pizza bites into your mouth or scoop up that sole remaining spoonful of mac 'n' cheese—don't do it! If you eat your child's food, either off his plate or as you prepare or clean up his meal, you might as well say, "Good-bye, skinny jeans. Hello, homely mom jeans!" (See Fat Habit #16.)

SLIM SOLUTION

There are three key reasons why this habit makes it almost impossible to eat a nutritious, balanced diet that promotes weight loss—even if your child's diet is relatively healthy.

1. | *Bite-size calories count.* Every little bite, morsel, or taste contains calories that most of us conveniently forget to count toward our daily total. What's worse, most moms do it repeatedly

during the day—we actually refer to it as "Mom's fourth meal." Many moms will find that when they stop doing this, they easily and quickly peel off some extra pounds. A food log can help you keep track of sneaky calories.

2. | *Kid foods lack what you need most.* Bread crusts, Cheerios, cheesy broccoli, chicken nuggets, cheese and crackers . . . they're not the most filling or nutritious options. They contain sugar and fat and pack a lot of calories to promote growth. While your kids may be able to spend the calories on these types of foods, you (and most other parents, for that matter) want and need foods that are a little harder-working, meaning their calories help fill you up so you stay satisfied longer. That means foods that are rich in fiber and/or protein. Put simply, a bowl of SpaghettiO's isn't going to cut it.

3. | *It's mindless noshing.* When you chow down while cleaning up, you usually do it mindlessly. On the other hand, when you sit down and eat off of your own plate using utensils, that's eating purposefully. There's a big difference. People who eat mindfully are more satisfied and consume fewer calories. In fact, research shows that mindless eaters take in twice as many calories before feeling satisfied compared with someone who eats purposefully.

How does being tuned in help you to slim down? When you eat mindlessly, the brain doesn't provide the correct signals to the stomach to signal when we're full. Think of it as the movie-theater-popcorn effect: We can plow through that ginormous bucket of popcorn—with only a few kernels and some greasy fingers to show for it—because we're so distracted by what's on the big screen.

The best fix for mindless munching is to keep a food log of everything you eat and drink for a week. In less than a week's time—if you're really honest—you'll see exactly where those crafty calories are creeping into your diet.

Other helpful tricks to avoid becoming a human garbage disposal: Chew gum when you're in the kitchen preparing meals or cleaning up to keep your mouth occupied. If you can't clean up without sneaking those last few scraps, ask your kids—if they're old enough—or partner to help clear the plates.

If you've tried all of these tricks and you still want those last few bites, get your own plate and utensils. Chances are, you won't want to go through the trouble. After all—do you really need another dirty dish to clean?

Still struggling to break your plate-picking habit? You may discover—with the help of your handy food log—that you're just not eating enough of your own meals and snacks during the day. Moms always make sure their little ones are well fed, but usually forget all about themselves. The solution: Stock up on quick snacks that provide balanced nutrition and satisfaction (aim for foods that contain protein and/or fiber, the two most filling nutrients), like fresh fruit or veggies with hummus or a yogurt-based dip. Some portable snack ideas that you can stash in your car, purse, or diaper bag include mixed nuts, dried fruit, or beef jerky. (For more of our favorite portable snacks, see Fat Habit #84, "I eat my way through the mall!")

FAT HABIT #19

My work is sucking all the energy out of me . . . and destroying my diet in the process. —JANET C.

The workplace is rife with weight-loss obstacles: looming layoffs, a badgering boss, vending machine munch breaks, a coworker's candy jar, business lunches, night shifts, travel, morning doughnuts—the list just keeps going.

We're working longer hours (traditional nine-to-five jobs have gone the way of guaranteed pension plans) and are on call more than ever during those dwindling "off" hours, thanks to technology. Companies are cutting costs and looking to squeeze as much as they can out of each employee. And in this sluggish economy, it can be difficult to find something better. These pressures mean more stress and less sleep for most of us—a dangerous combo that has been shown to trigger hunger hormones and cravings, making it harder for you to manage what you eat.

One of the biggest workplace hazards: on-the-job eating. Corporate America knows that making food easily available (with vending machines, an on-site cafeteria, and so on) means employees will log more time at work. While some office food options are getting healthier, baked goods, candy, soda, and other treats are still the most common picks at most places.

This is good for the company's bottom line but not yours—research from the Academy of Nutrition and Dietetics shows that more than a third of office workers are eating breakfast at their desks; as many as two-thirds regularly munch on lunch in their offices; nine in ten snack on the job; and 7 percent are even eating dinner desk-side. What's worse, we're shoving it in at record speed: The typical lunch hour has shrunk to just thirty-six minutes!

SLIM SOLUTIONS

We're both working women (some would say borderline workaholics) from New York City who have logged our share of seventy-hour workweeks, pulled a number of all-nighters, travel constantly, and have answered to some pretty horrible bosses! We know the constant struggles working women face to balance a healthy lifestyle with a career. Fortunately, we've compiled some of the best strategies to succeed at both.

SQUASH STRESS

This may seem like mission impossible, but these five easy tips will help you go from chaotic to centered.

1. | *Relax.* Consider yoga, meditation, visualization, or other coping mechanisms to deal with work stress.

2. | *Get more Z's.* Strive for one hour of sleep for every two hours that you are awake. For most adults, seven and a half hours of shut-eye a night should be a minimum.

3. | *Avoid drastic diets.* Going on a restrictive diet can also stimulate the release of cortisol and other stress hormones; instead, make small changes to your diet and focus on making healthful choices.

4. | *Take a break.* When you're out of the office, or even if you just need some downtime, turn on your out-of-office notification so you won't feel like you have to immediately respond to everyone.

5. | *Sneak in some activity.* Take ten or more minutes each day to get some physical activity. Exercise is one of the best ways to beat stress, and it will help you keep your resolve to eat healthier. If you can get outside, that's even better, because studies show that spending time outside is one of the best ways to reboot your brain.

LOBBY FOR WAIST MANAGEMENT

Ask your boss or human resource department about the possibility of offering healthier options at the office. For instance, instead of doughnuts and muffins at morning meetings, ask for a fruit bowl and/or low-fat yogurt. Gather a group of coworkers to add some heft to your request.

BROWN-BAG IT

Every meal eaten out or delivered to your desk ups your odds of being overweight, so it's important to limit the number of meals you eat out, preferably to no more than twice a week. Bring your own lunch from home; some good options include sandwiches on whole-grain bread, cups of broth-based soups, Greek yogurt and fruit, whole-grain veggie wraps, hummus with mixed veggies, and salads with lean protein.

When traveling, use Julie's trick: Make a quick stop at a nearby supermarket to pick up some fruit, yogurt, and nuts.

CREATE A HEALTHY SNACK STASH

Forget about chocolate and candy. Instead, stock your desk drawer with healthy snacks, such as dried fruit, individual packets of nuts, instant-oatmeal packets, and packets of Carnation Instant Breakfast or other protein shake mixes.

STUDY UP WHEN DINING OUT

Be sure to choose healthier options on the menu. (See Fat Habits #70, #71, and #72 on pages 174–84.) Get online and preview the nutrition information from the restaurant you're going to, and piece together a meal that has no more than 450 calories for breakfast, 500 calories for lunch, and 600 calories for dinner.

CHOOSE CAREFULLY AT THE CAFETERIA

When eating at the corporate cafeteria, head to the salad bar and pile on all the veggies you like. Top them off with a little lean protein (chicken, tuna, or eggs) to keep you satisfied. Veggie stir-fry, rice bowls, broth-based soups, and grilled chicken or fish options with whole-grain sides are all diet-friendly options.

WATCH THE CLOCK

Try to give yourself time to just eat—that means no computer, no texting, no buying items from Gilt.com or Overstock. Just sit there and eat. Focusing on your food will help you feel satisfied and cut back on calories.

FAT HABIT #20

My boss is psycho. . . . She's nice one day and mean to me the next. I'm so stressed out I'm eating more because of her. —KELLY D.

Workers today are riding the emotional roller coaster of the down economy, but add to that a boss who acts bipolar and it's no wonder you're craving comfort food to soothe the stress.

Everyone has either experienced or knows of someone who's had to work with a horrible boss—someone who praises you one day, then berates you the next. Stress that's out of your control—like traffic, unpredictable bosses, or an illness—is often the type of stress that wreaks the most havoc on your diet. Because we feel helpless we turn to quick comfort—whether that's a chocolate bar, a brownie, or booze.

SLIM SOLUTIONS

When work stress starts to impact your life away from work, leaves you preoccupied, and adversely impacts your physical and emotional health and well-being, it's time to take serious steps to improve your work life or start looking for a new job.

All anyone can ask of you is to do your best: If you're doing that, don't worry about what your boss has to say about your work. Raise your concerns and document incidents of mistreatment to human resources, and if they're no help, take all the necessary steps to cover your own butt. For example, document e-mails where your boss may ask for one thing, then another. Keep a file of e-mail correspondence where she's been out of line with you so that you have everything documented.

TAKE CARE OF NUMERO UNO

Start paying attention to your physical and emotional health by logging how you're feeling in your food journal. Believe us, the better your diet and the more you can stick with daily exercise, the more you'll be able to handle at work and the less overwhelmed and stressful the situation will seem.

BEAT STRESS WITH HEALTHIER HABITS

Here are some healthier solutions for when work stress strikes:

Talk to someone: Sharing your feelings is one way to help you manage stress and come up with a solution. A psychologist is a great spend during rough times, but venting to a friend also helps you get your head clear on what you need to do for yourself.

Do at least one thing daily that you love. If that's eating chocolate-chip cookies, make it something healthier, like walking your dog, taking a bath, reading a book.

Give thanks: Every day, tell yourself what you have in your life that you're thankful for. Do this in the morning, before you even get to the office, to help reframe your mind to help you cope with your work situation.

FAT HABIT #21

*My boyfriend [husband, lover, or significant other]
loves my curves more than I do!* —RACHEL M.

It's not uncommon for men to embrace a woman's curves—it's natural biology. Studies consistently show that for the most part, men will find a woman who is at a healthy weight more attractive than one who's underweight. (There's no denying that Kim Kardashian, Beyoncé, and Jennifer Lopez have made curves a hot commodity.)

However, this may interfere with your desire to slim down. Perhaps he's constantly trying to get you to eat fatty foods or skip your workouts. It's important to know why he prefers a plumper partner. For instance, if your significant other is carrying around a few extra pounds himself, he may not want you to lose weight because it would make him feel bad about himself. Or it may be fear: He may be worried that you're going to get rid of him, or that you're trying to lose weight to look more attractive to someone else. Once you know what's behind his behavior, you can address it in a positive way.

SLIM SOLUTIONS

SHOW HIM SOME LOVE

Some partners feel threatened or insecure when their loved one starts to lose weight, exercise more, and/or swap out bad behaviors for new, healthier habits. If you sense this is going on, giving your guy attention and plenty of love can help reassure him that you are trying to lose weight only for your own health and wellness, and that you have no intention of leaving him. Men respond well to praise, but when it comes to criticism, not so much. Try to keep the communication positive, and bite your tongue if you feel you want to say something critical.

SOLVE DIET DISCORD

The number-one rule to slim down and stay in love is: Never nag, beg, bribe, or coerce your partner into changing, says Cynthia Sass, MPH, MA, RD, CSSD, author of the *New York Times* bestselling book *S.A.S.S! Yourself Slim: Conquer Cravings, Drop Pounds, and Lose Inches.* "You can't make someone want to change; pushing will only backfire and can hurt your communication and trust."

EXPLAIN YOUR INTENTIONS

If you're trying to eat healthfully and your partner isn't ready or willing to join you, take the time to let him or her know what you're doing, why it's important to you, how you expect it to impact how you eat together, and what you need from him or her, Sass says. Make it clear that you may need to alter how you eat together, such as getting takeout from two different places, or customizing your meals by sharing some but not all of the ingredients. If your hubby wants to eat a stuffed burrito, make yourself a healthy taco salad of greens tossed with pico de gallo, topped with black beans, roasted corn, and sliced avocado—hold the tortilla, rice, meat, cheese, and sour cream, she says.

LEAD BY EXAMPLE

If your partner isn't on board, the best thing you can do is let him or her see how great you feel and how much you're enjoying your new way of eating, Sass says. Offer bites or tastes of your healthy meals and snacks, but don't make it a bone of contention, and avoid being an evangelist—enthusiasm often comes across as judgment, even if that's not your intention, she says. Most likely, your partner will come around; when you see someone close to you feeling happier and healthier, it can be highly contagious.

FAT HABIT #22

My husband shows he loves me with the treats he brings home for me. I don't want to say something and hurt his feelings.

—JEANNIE O.

It's an equation that many of us know and use in our own lives. It's how moms show children they love them, and it's something many of us carry on as adults. Think about holidays, birthdays, celebrations, and other get-togethers where food and treats are an expression of love.

SLIM SOLUTION

The solution for this is relatively simple: Gently ask your partner to show his love for you with good-for-you goodies going forward. But before you do that, cushion the blow by acknowledging that you appreciate his gifts. Then you can explain why you want to eat better and that it would make you very happy if he could help you with your goals. You can work together to come up with ideas that won't derail your diet.

Some of our clients have even given their loved ones lists of things that they'd appreciate in place of treats. They've included exercise equipment and apparel, healthy cooking gadgets and appliances, personal trainer sessions or gym memberships, and cooking classes and healthy cookbooks.

FAT HABIT #23

My friends' unhealthy habits have rubbed off on me. —SARA P.

Is obesity contagious, much like a virus? That's what some researchers have suggested in recent years. However, what seems to be more likely: The clustering of obesity stems from both biological traits (genetics among siblings) as well as behavioral factors that are shared among those in your social network, including your spouse and friends.

Being overweight and obese are considered "socially contagious" because people within social networks share many of the same beliefs and tend to adopt similar habits and lifestyles, knowingly and unknowingly. Of course, this could be for better, but more often it's for worse. In a landmark Harvard Medical School study that was published in the *New England Journal of Medicine* in 2007, researchers tracked more than twelve thousand health care professionals for thirty-two years. They found that obesity risk was:

- 57 percent greater if your close friend is obese
- 40 percent greater if a sibling is obese
- 37 percent greater if a spouse is obese

What's striking about these results is that same-sex friends have more influence over our body weight than siblings, suggesting that our behaviors are more important than our genes.

A more recent study from Arizona State University published in the *American Journal of Public Health* reaffirmed these findings. The ASU researchers examined 101 women ages 25 to 45 years old, and nearly a thousand of their family and friends. By looking at the participants' body mass index (BMI), they found that women are more likely to be obese if their peers are overweight or obese. In fact, women who had someone in their social network who was overweight or obese were 59 percent more likely to be overweight or obese themselves, and this effect was strongest among friends who were the closest. They also found that same-sex relationships impact our body weight more than those with the opposite sex do.

There are many theories as to why our friends (primarily same-sex pals) have such an impact on our weight. Some of the effects are thought to be subliminal, so you're not even aware of them. For example, if your friends are overweight, it makes it easier to accept your weight, even if it's more than what you'd like to weigh.

Your eating and exercise habits may also be impacted by what your friends want to eat and do socially. Overweight friends may want to go out to eat more often and are less likely to recommend going for a jog, hike, or swim. Think about it: What do you do socially with your friends? Do you socialize after a sweat session, chatting about what healthy foods you're going to eat? Or do you go out for margaritas and burritos at the local Mexican restaurant and swap stories about the latest office gossip?

SLIM SOLUTIONS

While we want to accept our friends as they are (no matter their size), we need to be aware that we may be subconsciously adopting their behaviors. You can lose weight without unfriending anyone by using these tips:

SHARE THE WEALTH

After reading this book, pass it along to a pal who you think can use it most. Then tell her to pass it along to her closest friend. Just as unhealthy behaviors are contagious, healthy ones can be too.

MAKE SOME NEW "FRIENDS"

Visit our website, AppforHealth.com, where we provide daily inspiration to our online friends. Other sites we like include Spark People.com, WeightWatchers.com, Active.com, Livestrong.com, and Curves.com. Stop by to read the information and posts, or use Facebook and Twitter to get news feeds from healthy "friends" like registered dietitians and fitness trainers. Online health and nutrition tools can help you get a different weight perspective.

RECRUIT RECEPTIVE PALS

Have a discussion with family members or friends who you think would be open to adopting healthier behaviors with you.

EXPAND YOUR CIRCLE

Join a health club, or a local hiking, cycling, or other activity-oriented club, where you'll be more likely to meet individuals who share your desire to be healthy and active.

FAT HABIT #24

I finally got a boyfriend, but I've gained 6 pounds since we started dating. I can't continue on the pound-per-month plan anymore!
—CAROL G.

There's a lot to love about your new sweetie—but those extra pounds that you've put on since meeting him isn't one of them. Research shows that males, whether we're living with, dating, or married to them, make it harder for us to maintain our weight.

After studying nearly 1,300 couples, researchers at the University of North Carolina reported that women who live with or marry a man double or triple their risk for becoming obese. Men in couples gain too, but women typically gain more. And the longer you are with a partner, the heavier you're likely to become. Interestingly enough, if a woman becomes single again, she tends to lose weight—there's a reason why they call it a "divorce diet."

SLIM SOLUTIONS

There's no need to say sayonara to your significant other. The solution: Simply be aware of the negative weight effects of being in a relationship. Whether you're slacking off because you feel comfortable, settled, and secure or you've picked up some of his bad habits, you can get back on track with these five slim-single-girl rules:

PRETEND YOU'RE STILL AVAILABLE

Take a good look at yourself and ask whether you would be comfortable trying to date. Keep a stash of single-girl apparel that makes you look and feel great, and wear it at least once a month to make sure it still fits.

DON'T EAT HIS FOOD

You and your new love are so close that you're starting to dress alike, and you can even finish his sentences. This closeness may be great for your relationship, but it can spell disaster for your diet. The solution: Make sure to keep your own diet identity. Stick to a healthy diet and follow our meal plans in Chapter 7. If he's a meat-and-potatoes guy and you want to have what he's having on occasion, make sure to enjoy a smaller portion.

LET YOUR APPETITE BE YOUR GUIDE

To ensure that you're eating because you're truly physiologically hungry and not simply because your man is hungry, use the Hunger Scale (on page 39). This handy tool will help you get back to eating according to your body's needs, not his.

MAKE YOUR HOME HEALTHY

If you live with your man, make sure it's a "clean-eating" environment. Set some ground rules with him about the types of food that you want in your kitchen (healthy fruits, vegetables, and whole grains), and if he brings home junk food, make sure it's out of sight and reach for you. Take a healthy cooking course (by yourself or together) if you need to brush up on some leaner cooking techniques.

LIMIT CUDDLE TIME ON THE COUCH

Research shows that limiting the amount of time you spend in front of the TV to no more than two hours a day can significantly improve your diet and eating habits. TV watching often goes hand in hand with treats and junk food. If you're not in front of the TV, you may be out exercising or doing something that's more productive. Do you really need to watch another episode of *NCIS* or a not-so-realistic reality show?

FAT HABIT #25

*I just started a new job and my colleagues want to meet for drinks . . .
like three nights a week! I don't want to feel like the odd one out.*

—SARA S.

You may think you don't have a whole lot of options here. You could skip it, but you don't want to be left out, especially as the new girl. You could go, but you don't want to be the only person not partying. What's a girl to do?

SLIM SOLUTIONS

We have lots of experience in this area: Katherine suffers from migraines if she drinks, so she skips sipping, and Julie is a teetotaler, for no good reason other than the fact that it's easier for her to manage her calories when she doesn't drink. Check out some of our tried-and-true tips:

ARRIVE LATE AND LEAVE EARLY

When meeting friends or coworkers for drinks or dinner, try to arrive a little late. This way you can skip the martini at the bar before dinner. You can also head out if and when the temptation of tequila and tortilla chips becomes too much to bear. (Of course, if you find it's too hard to go and not drink or indulge, you have every right to pass on the plans altogether.) Here are some excuses we've used to get out of a cocktail convention:

I'm taking care of my friends' dog.
I have guests coming to visit and have to get my apartment ready.
Oh . . . I ate such a late lunch, I won't be hungry.
I've got _____ (track, swimming, CrossFit) practice to go to tonight.
I'm hosting _____ (book, dinner, investment) club this month.

LIMIT YOURSELF

Alcohol in small amounts is actually okay and can be good for your heart, but it's not terribly diet-friendly. Alcohol makes it hard to manage your weight because it adds empty calories to your diet. A 5-ounce glass of wine has 120 calories, while a serving of hard liquor (1½ ounces) has 110 calories. That might not seem too bad, but beware: These drinks are often served in oversize glasses that double or triple the calories. Plus, alcohol stimulates your appetite and it reduces your inhibitions. If you want to sip but are also interested in slimming down, keep it to no more than four to five drinks per week and plan accordingly.

SUGGEST A CHANGE OF PLANS

Instead of always meeting friends for drinks after work, make plans to take a CrossFit, Spin, or Zumba class, or go for a speed walk, suggests Martha McKittrick, RD, CDE (www.citygirlbites.com), a registered dietitian and certified diabetes educator. You can then grab a healthy dinner afterward—minus the alcohol. Or suggest meeting for coffee or even lunch (there's less of a chance for cocktails at a midday meal).

SIP SLOWLY

It's simple, but it works: The slower you drink, the less alcohol you'll consume, McKittrick says. How to slow your sipping? Drink a type of alcohol that's meant to be savored. For example, red wine often goes down more slowly than white wine. Or opt for a stronger beverage, like Scotch, which takes a little longer to drink. Try having a glass of water, club soda, or other calorie-free beverage in between cocktails to help pace yourself, she suggests.

AVOID AUTO-REFILL

If you're at a function where someone is constantly refilling drinks, remain on high alert and subtly cover your glass so it doesn't get refilled.

VISUALIZE SUCCESS

Imagine the scenario before heading out to meet friends or colleagues: Picture them offering you a drink and see yourself politely refusing. Set your goal as to how many drinks you will have before going out, and stay focused on sticking with it, she suggests.

FAT HABIT #26

I noticed that ever since I joined Pinterest,
I've gained 8 pounds.

—RACHEL D.

Red Velvet and Nutella Cake in a Jar, Santa Hat Brownies, Chicken Taco Chili, Oreo Layer Dessert, Chocolate–Peanut Butter Parfaits, Frozen Strawberry Mojitos, Easy-Peasy Cherry Cheese Cobbler, Ale and Cheddar Soup . . .

We think Pinterest should come with a warning: "Pinterest will make you hungry . . . and maybe even fat!"

If you're not familiar with Pinterest, it's a virtual scrapbooking site that has become the most popular social networking site after Twitter and Facebook. It has millions of users, mostly women. The basic idea: You "grab" and "pin" images that you like from the Web and post them onto personal pinboards.

So what does Pinterest have to do with extra pounds? The most popular Pinterest topics include food and beverage, and not surprisingly, the more popular pins are generally the most glorious, delicious, decadent, mouthwatering appetizers, main dishes, desserts, and drinks known to mankind. These images are so irresistible that you'll likely drool on your keyboard.

SLIM SOLUTIONS

We both use Pinterest, and Appetite for Health has its own Pinterest page, but when we're on the site, we try to focus on images that help us improve our diet, not destroy it.

You're already exposed to so many unhealthy foods in real life; you don't need to make things worse by salivating over virtual images of so-good-I-swear-they're-calling-my-name calorie bombs. Research shows that people who struggle the most with their weight are much more susceptible to their environment. Use the following pinning pointers to create a healthy online environment for yourself:

DELETE YOUR DECADENT PINS AND PINBOARDS

Delete your pinboards or pins that include your most physique-damaging food images and recipes. You don't need recipes for the "Fluffiest Chocolate-Chip Cookie Recipe—Ever" or "Nutella Fudge." If the pin comes from boards called "Mmmmmm," "Goodies," "Yumminess," or "Heaven on Earth," chances are it's not a waist-friendly recipe.

GET MOTIVATED

Create new pinboards that serve as healthy inspirations. We like those that feature quotes that help keep us motivated to move and eat right. Some of our favorite words of wisdom:

"Junk food that you have been craving for an hour or the body you have wanted for years? It's your choice."

"Remember: Fat lasts longer than flavor."

"If you give up today, think about how you'll feel a month from now when you could be 5 pounds lighter."

SIMPLIFY SEARCHING

You can search the site using hashtags, as with Twitter, so use #healthyrecipes, #nutrition, #fitness, #abs, #getfit, or #wholeliving to start creating better-for-you boards.

MAKE NUMBERS A NECESSITY

Repin only those recipes that have nutritional analyses. As a general rule, if a recipe is from a nonnutrition source and it doesn't provide any nutrition information, it's probably not good for you.

PIN FROM THE PROS

Follow us, and other dietitians, like Ellie Krieger or Michelle Dudash. We also follow pinboards from Skinnytaste, Skinny Kitchen, *Cooking Light*, and *EatingWell*.

FAT HABIT #27

I don't think I've gained weight. . . . I wear the same jeans size as when I was a senior in high school. —JOCELYN G.

If you're still wearing the same jeans size as when Madonna was known as the "Material Girl," you rock. We also hate to be the bearers of bad news, but don't feel too smug.

These days there is rampant inflation in the sizing of women's and men's clothes. It's referred to in the industry as "vanity sizing." And you guessed it: Manufacturers are putting smaller size numbers on larger-size clothes, in an effort to make you feel great about wearing the same jeans or dress size you did twenty years ago.

A study of dresses dating found that the same-size woman would have worn a size-fourteen dress from the 1937 Sears catalog. By 1967 clothing standards, she would have worn an eight, and today that same-size woman would wear a zero dress size. So while the label on your jeans may still say size four, six, or eight, that doesn't mean you haven't gained weight since your yearbook picture was taken.

And not only are today's sizes roomier than those from just a few years ago, but different designers have varying definitions of sizes. If you are "mostly" a size six, we bet you have a few size eights, fours, and perhaps even some twos in your closet. In a 2003 study, researchers measured a thousand pairs of women's pants and found as much as an 8½-inch variation in the waist of a size four.

SLIM SOLUTION

While it may be a great boost to your self-esteem to fit into a pair of size-six jeans, you can forget judging your actual size according to what the clothing label says.

Instead, rely on the scale (see Fat Habit #59, "I can't stand to weigh myself"), and take your waist, bust, and hip measurements with a tape measure. And if all the crazy sizing has *you* going crazy, try using a body measurement technology like the one at Me-Ality (www.me-ality.com). This free service helps you get accurate sizing (it takes more than 200,000 measurements!), so you'll know what size you'll fit into from a variety of designers.

I THOUGHT I *WAS* DIETING

FEELING WEIGHED DOWN BY TOO MUCH WEIGHT-LOSS INFORMA-
tion? If the sheer amount of information out there isn't enough to
get you to throw your fork down in frustration, perhaps the fact
that a lot of it is conflicting might be. One day experts tell you to
cut out carbs; the next day they advise forgoing fat. A study finds
that three square meals is your ticket to slimming down; shortly
after, another suggests more frequent mini-meals is the key. Sure,
nutrition knowledge is power, but if you spend too much time trying to stay abreast of the latest dieting research, it's easy to lose track
of the real skinny: What really counts is not the latest fad, but what
you do (or don't do!) every day.

If you know some of the more common "diet" mistakes people
make, you can sidestep them and stay on track. Read on to learn
which myths could be making you fat, and smart solutions to avoid
these traps.

FAT HABIT #28

I try all the latest diets and nothing ever seems to work.

—CHRISTEN B.

Nutrition fiction is everywhere. You may expect it from infomercials, but your local newspaper or favorite magazine? It's true—you can find big fat diet lies on the pages of these periodicals. With promises of quick fixes with no effort, it's no wonder that trendy fasts and fad diets that make for splashy headlines are so popular. And yet the United States is *still* the fattest nation on earth.

Why? Many of these weight-loss techniques can actually lead you down the path of deprivation, which often results in weight loss, followed by regain. Others are outright harmful, depriving your body of important nutrients, or worse.

SLIM SOLUTIONS

USE COMMON SENSE

"Lose 15 pounds in a week." "Drop a size in two days." "Shed pounds without diet or exercise." If it sounds too good to be true, it probably is! Many fraudsters know how desperate people are to look slim and sexy. Don't fall for their tricks. And trust us: It can happen to anyone. We know many well-educated people who've fallen prey to diet scams.

ASK THE RIGHT QUESTIONS

The next time you hear diet advice, ask yourself the following questions:

* *What are the credentials of the person offering advice? Is he or she a "real" expert?* Registered dietitians, RDs, are the real

nutrition pros. To earn their credentials, they must receive a minimum of a bachelor's degree in nutrition from a college or university, complete nine hundred hours in a supervised practice program, and pass a national examination administered by the Commission on Dietetic Registration. To maintain this registration, dietitians complete ongoing continuing-education requirements. Other credible nutrition credentials include PhDs, MPHs, and MDs who specialize in nutrition science.

- *Is this person selling supplements or pills that must be taken or used in combination with his or her diet?* Unless the supplement is backed by nutrition research substantiating the need for a specific nutrient, or you have a medical condition requiring supplementation, pass on the pill! Most people don't need a daily vitamin or mineral supplement. Ask why a supplement or pill is necessary and what research this person has to support his or her claims.

- *Does the diet require omitting whole food groups (like carbohydrates)? Do specific foods need to be eaten daily?* Balanced nutrition and healthy weight loss allow for variety and moderation. Prohibiting whole food groups decreases your intake of vitamins and minerals and is unnecessary for weight loss.

- *Does this person use testimonials ("My last client lost 20 pounds in two weeks!") rather than nutrition research to substantiate his or her diet or supplement claims?* Nutrition science is based on research, which means it has been subjected to the rigors of multiple studies and reviewed by other scientists. In other words, findings of scientific studies are usually valid and trustworthy. Anecdotal evidence is not enough proof that a plan or pill works.

- *Does he or she promise quick, dramatic results rather than long-*

term success? It's a simple fact: Sustainable weight loss takes time. "Guaranteed" speedy results should be a red flag that you may be dealing with a quack.

Seek credible sources of nutrition and diet information. If you're reading this book, congratulations! You've come to the right place for sound nutrition and diet info. All of the weight-loss advice on these pages is provided by registered dietitians and is based on peer-reviewed, published scientific studies.

You can find an RD in your area by checking with the Academy of Nutrition and Dietetics—www.eatright.org—or calling their Consumer Nutrition Hotline at: 1-800-366-1655.

FAT HABIT #29

I'm always going up and down in weight. I'm a yo-yo dieter.

—ALICIA N.

You know the vicious cycle: Lose weight on a diet. Come off diet and gain weight (and a few extra pounds) again. Repeat.

Are repeated diets making us fatter? According to some obesity experts, the answer is *yes*. Their research suggests that going on a "diet" is not the answer to the nation's obesity problem. For many overweight people, habitual dieting only makes their weight woes worse. That's because most people can't sustain a diet that cuts out favorite foods or slashes too many calories. As soon as you come off the plan, the weight piles on again—and in many cases, you end up tipping the scales even more than when you first started.

It's not just a matter of weak willpower. Some findings suggest that dieters who have regained weight may be struggling against biological mechanisms that make them regain weight and feel hungry more readily than people who never dieted in the first place.

This pound rebound may be caused in part by your hormones kicking in, making you feel hungrier. Leptin, the feel-full hormone, tends to fall after weight loss, according to research. The result: Appetite increases and metabolism slows. One study indicates that one year after a weight-loss diet, leptin levels among the study subjects were still one-third lower than they were at the start of the study. Other hormones that stimulate hunger, in particular ghrelin, whose levels increased with weight loss, made the subjects' appetites stronger than they were at the study outset.

Does this mean you're destined for diet failure? Not at all. Permanent weight loss *is* possible! Despite the challenges that may result from years of yo-yo dieting, "overweight" doesn't have to be your fate. The fact is, diets that involve cutting calories usually work. But the big caveat is that you have to be able to stick to it for the long haul. As we tell our clients, whatever it is that you do to lose weight, you have to *keep doing it* to make sure it stays off! *The main challenge is this: You must cut calories without going hungry.* And to do this, you must eat smarter! We can definitely help you become a smarter eater.

SLIM SOLUTIONS

EAT MORE TO WEIGH LESS

How can you cut calories while simultaneously adding foods to your diet? Believe it or not, **the healthiest, smartest weight-loss strategies often require *adding* foods to your diet!** But, of course, you have to add the right kinds of foods.

Which foods are they? Those with a high water and fiber content, like broth-based soups and fruits and vegetables. "A key to avoiding hunger while managing calories is to eat foods that offer a satisfying portion in fewer calories," says Barbara Rolls, PhD, professor of nutritional sciences at Penn State University, and author of *The Ultimate Volumetrics Diet: Smart, Simple, Science-Based Strategies for Losing Weight and Keeping It Off.* "Fruits, vegetables, and soup have water and that provides volume with no calories." Basically, you're pumping up the volume of your foods without pumping up your calorie intake.

Experts refer to these types of foods as "low energy density" (LED) foods. Energy density is the amount of energy—or calories—in a particular weight of food. For the same number of calories, a person can consume a larger portion of an LED food than a food that has a higher energy density.

Aim to get more high-volume LED foods (see list below for ideas) into your diet. Start with the recommended five-plus servings of fruits and vegetables each day. That may sound like a lot, but you're actually hitting two goals at once: You'll meet your daily fiber mark and you'll be feeling more satisfied from the volume of food.

VERY LOW-DENSITY FOODS INCLUDE:

- Nonstarchy vegetables
- Nonfat milk
- Fruits
- Soup broths

VERY HIGH-DENSITY FOODS INCLUDE:

- Crackers
- Chips
- Cookies
- Chocolate/Candies
- Butter

When you start filling your diet with low energy density foods, you'll find they crowd out the fattier, less healthy picks, which can lead to overeating.

DON'T SKIP MEALS

Yo-yo dieting is often a result of skipping meals, which only leaves you feeling hungry and deprived. As you probably are well aware, deprivation spells disaster for your diet (and incidentally sets you up for another round of yo-yoing). Instead, eat meals and snacks at regular intervals.

PUMP UP PROTEIN

Protein can also help you put an end to roller-coaster dieting. The nutrient is more satisfying than carbohydrates or fats, and may be the secret weapon in weight control. Meals that are higher in protein can help reduce hunger and increase your sense of fullness. Higher-protein diets, those containing approximately 18 to 35 percent of daily calorie intake, can keep you full for longer.

Your goal: **Eat protein at every meal—and especially at breakfast.** Recent research has shown that starting your day with eggs or another protein-packed breakfast food can cut your total calorie intake for the day.

Obesity experts believe that the quality of protein—rather than the quantity—may be more important when it comes to enhancing satiety while dialing down hunger hormones.

While the jury is still out on how much protein is best, we suggest at least 20 grams of high-quality protein for breakfast as a start.

High-Protein Snacks Under 200 Calories

Almonds

1 ounce (23 almonds) provides 170 calories, 6 grams of protein, 3.5 grams of fiber, 75 milligrams of calcium, and 7.4 milligrams of vitamin E (the most of all nuts), as well as antioxidants and heart-healthy fats.

Cereal with milk and fruit

A whole-grain cereal paired with low-fat milk and fresh fruit provides carbohydrates and protein, along with vitamins and minerals. Choose a cereal that has at least 3 grams of fiber per serving. Top with fresh fruit.

Fresh fruit paired with low-fat cheese

Apple or pear slices with a couple of ounces of reduced-fat cheese.

Peanut butter sandwich

Peanut butter on whole-grain bread is a high-energy, tasty, portable snack. Peanut butter has heart-healthy fat and is high in protein.

Pistachios

1 ounce of pistachios is 49 nuts—the most nuts per serving. It's low in calories, with 160, and it's high in fiber, vitamin B6, and the phytonutrients lutein and zeaxanthin.

Popcorn sprinkled with Parmesan

Low-fat microwave popcorn is a whole-grain snack; when sprinkled with 2 tablespoons of grated Parmesan, this snack adds protein and 120 milligrams of calcium.

Trail mix

The key to this healthy snack is keeping the portions in check and opting for one that contains dried fruit, nuts, seeds, and whole-grain cereal. Avoid trail mix with candy pieces, to reduce fat.

7 Foods That Help You Fill Up—Not Out

1. **Broth-Based Soups**. Start off with soup! "Broth-based soups can contribute to a feeling of fullness, and can keep you from overindulging during the main course or dessert," says Dr. Rolls. Soups like miso or chicken noodle are most effective; heavy, cream-based soups, such as New England clam chowder or cream of anything, may help fill you up, but they also come at a high calorie cost. And keep in mind that soup isn't only a cold-weather food. In the summer, try chilled gazpacho or cold cucumber soup.

2. **Beans and Legumes**. Beans and legumes have a lot going for them— they're tasty, versatile, nutritious, and filling. Since beans can add up to a lot of calories if you eat more than a serving or two, it's a good idea to combine them with vegetables that are low in calories and will also help to keep you feeling full longer. Beans and legumes also have a great added perk—they are inexpensive.

3. **Nuts**. It's okay to get a little nutty—while nuts are energy-dense and high in fat (though it's the healthy kind), their protein content can keep you feeling full and often stave off a binge later in the day. We suggest having nuts with a glass of water. The volume that water adds to the stomach combined with the slow-to-digest nuts makes this a perfect quickie fill-up. Not to mention that being hydrated can help with hunger management.

4. **Chicken**. When it's baked, grilled, or broiled, chicken is a great source of protein. Fish, lean meat, tofu, and other proteins, like beans, legumes, and eggs, are also terrific—chicken just has a bit of a leg up because it's so widely available, inexpensive, and easy to incorporate into meals.

5. **Fruits and Veggies**. This dynamic duo is probably one of the best weight-loss weapons in your arsenal. High in fiber and water, they'll fill you up without blowing your calorie budget. Aim for five to nine servings every day. Find fun and creative ways to incorporate them into

your diet: You can snack on them, add them to recipes, or make them the star of the meal (like a salad).

6. **Eggs**. There are about a dozen reasons to love eggs—for one, the high-quality protein in eggs helps you to feel full longer and stay energized. In one study published in the *Journal of the American College of Nutrition*, researchers found that having eggs for breakfast helped overweight adults feel more full and consume an average of 330 fewer calories throughout the day than adults who ate a bagel-based breakfast that contained the same number of calories.

7. **Nonfat or Low-fat Greek Yogurt**. Nonfat or low-fat Greek yogurt is thicker than regular yogurt and contains more protein per serving (up to 23 grams per cup). Note: It does contain slightly less calcium. Top with fresh fruit and enjoy!

FAT HABIT #30

The only diet that works for me is the no-carb diet. I can't even look at carbs if I want to lose weight! —AMBER W.

Poor carbs—the much-maligned nutrient has been taking the blame for our weight woes for far too long. In fact, the idea that carbs are mainly to blame for the obesity crisis is one of the most enduring diet myths out there.

We're here to do some damage control for carbs. Our body actually needs carbs—they're the main source of energy in our diet. It's when we overeat carbs (or really any nutrient, for that matter) that we run into trouble. Plus, cutting out carbs entirely is too restrictive, and restrictive diets just don't last. Studies show that it's common to regain lost weight, regardless of the diet plan, particularly if it's too restrictive to live with permanently.

SLIM SOLUTION

CHOOSE GOOD CARBS OVER *NO* CARBS.

To lose weight and keep it off, you don't have to cut out all or even most carbs. Carbohydrates are found in a wide variety of foods— from healthy, protein-rich choices like Greek yogurt to nutrient-poor, calorie-rich foods and beverages like desserts, table sugar, soda, and other sweetened beverages. What's important is that you choose healthy carbohydrates that bring nutrients and fiber with them.

This means whole grains (the less processed, the better), vegetables, fruits, and beans. Skip the easily digested carbohydrates from refined grains—white bread, white rice, and the like—as well as pastries, sugared sodas, and other highly processed foods, because these *may* contribute to weight gain, interfere with weight loss, and promote diabetes and heart disease.

FAT HABIT #31

I think that eating fat is what's making me fat.
So I just don't eat it. —KELLY Z.

Forgoing fat? That's *so* 1985! Once upon a time, people believed that to get skinny, they had to cut out all the fat from their diet. Low- and no-fat diets were especially popular in the 1980s and 1990s—entire cookbooks, television shows, and magazine articles were devoted to the low-fat craze.

This fat fixation did have some merit. One of the main beefs people had with beef and other fatty foods: Fat has about twice as many calories per gram as carbohydrates and protein. A gram of fat has 9 calories, while a gram of carbohydrate or protein has just 4 calories. That means you could eat twice as much carbohydrate or protein as fat for the same number of calories.

Cholesterol Check

Cholesterol isn't a fat—it's a waxy, fatlike substance. Your body manufactures some cholesterol, and it also absorbs dietary cholesterol from foods of animal origin, such as meat and eggs. Cholesterol is vital because, among other important functions, it helps build your body's cells and produces certain hormones. But your body makes enough cholesterol to meet its needs—you don't need any extra dietary cholesterol.

Excessive dietary cholesterol, as you may know, can increase your unhealthy LDL (low-density lipoprotein) cholesterol level. This can increase your risk of heart disease and stroke.

It wasn't just a weight worry with fat—there were some health concerns surrounding the nutrient as well. Saturated and trans fats can raise cholesterol levels in the blood, increasing your risk for heart disease. These fats also may play a role in other diseases, including obesity and cancer. Plus, some fatty foods (think greasy wings, French fries, and rich desserts) often have fewer vitamins and minerals than low-fat foods. And then there's new research about the possible dangers and benefits of dietary fats (sometimes called fatty acids).

As with carbs, it's not necessarily the *quantity* of fat in your diet, but the *quality* of fat you consume that matters most.

SLIM SOLUTION

HAVE SOME FAT TO GET SKINNY

Fat is essential to your health because it supports a number of your body's functions. Some vitamins, for instance, must have fat to dissolve and nourish your body. And lest we forget—it also adds texture and flavor to food! Don't nix all fat from your diet.

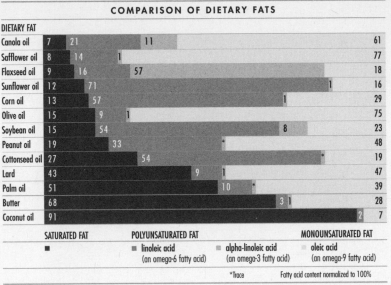

COMPARISON OF DIETARY FATS

DIETARY FAT	SATURATED FAT	POLYUNSATURATED FAT — linoleic acid (an omega-6 fatty acid)	alpha-linoleic acid (an omega-3 fatty acid)	MONOUNSATURATED FAT — oleic acid (an omega-9 fatty acid)
Canola oil	7	21	11	61
Safflower oil	8	14	1	77
Flaxseed oil	9	16	57	18
Sunflower oil	12	71	1	16
Corn oil	13	57	1	29
Olive oil	15	9	1	75
Soybean oil	15	54	8	23
Peanut oil	19	33	*	48
Cottonseed oil	27	54	*	19
Lard	43	9	1	47
Palm oil	51	10	*	39
Butter	68	3	1	28
Coconut oil	91	2		7

*Trace   Fatty acid content normalized to 100%

Source: POS Pilot Plant Corporation

KNOW YOUR FATS

The key to a healthy diet is to choose foods that contain more "good fats" than "bad fats" and that are free of trans fat. "Good" fats—also known as monounsaturated and polyunsaturated fats—lower disease risk. "Bad" fats—saturated and especially trans fats—increase disease risk. Foods high in good fats include vegetable oils (such as olive, canola, sunflower, soy, and corn), nuts, seeds, and fish. Foods high in bad fats include red meat, butter, cheese, and ice cream, as well as processed foods made with trans fat from partially hydrogenated oil.

And keep in mind that foods contain different types of fats at varying levels. For example, butter contains unsaturated fats, but a large percentage of the total fat is saturated fat. And canola oil has a high percentage of monounsaturated fat but also contains smaller amounts of polyunsaturated and saturated fat. Take a look

Coconut Oil: Is It All It's Cracked Up to Be?

Coconut oil, which has a slightly different makeup from other oils, has been touted to help with everything from weight loss to Alzheimer's disease. There are few solid studies (and by this, we mean peer-reviewed clinical trials published in reputable journals) looking at the effect of coconut oil on human health.

Coconut oil is unusual in that it contains a type of fat known as medium-chain triglycerides (MCTs). Some researchers have claimed that because MCTs are metabolized differently from other fats, they could offer some health benefits, particularly for slimming down. However, weight-loss studies using coconut oil have shown little to "modest" (about 4 pounds lost over four months) weight-loss results. Other studies looking at coconut oil for the treatment of heart disease and Alzheimer's have not produced successful outcomes. **The bottom line: Don't go nuts for coconut oil. There is no good evidence behind any of the recent health claims.**

at the chart on page 84 to see some common sources of fat and the breakdown of each.

DO SOME MATH TO GET THE RIGHT FIX OF FAT

Need help calculating what your daily fat intake should be in grams? Multiply your daily total calorie intake by the recommended percentage of fat intake. Divide that total by 9, which is the number of calories in a gram of fat. For example, here's how a saturated fat limit of 7 percent looks if you eat 1,600 calories a day. Multiply 1,600 by 0.07 to get 112 calories. Divide 112 by 9 to get about 12 grams of saturated fat.

USDA RECOMMENDATIONS FOR
DIETARY FAT AND CHOLESTEROL INTAKE

TYPE OF FAT	RECOMMENDATION	MAJOR FOOD SOURCES
Total fat	This includes all types of dietary fat. Limit total fat intake to 20 to 35 percent of your daily calories. Based on a 2,000-calorie-a-day diet, this amounts to about 44 to 78 grams of total fat a day.	Plant- and animal-based foods.
Monounsaturated fat	While no specific amount is recommended, the USDA guidelines advise eating foods rich in this healthy fat while staying within your total fat allowance.	Olive oil, peanut oil, canola oil, avocados, poultry, nuts, and seeds.
Polyunsaturated fat	While no specific amount is recommended, the guidelines advise eating foods rich in this healthy fat while staying within your total fat allowance.	Vegetable oils (such as safflower, corn, sunflower, soy, and cottonseed oils), nut oils (such as peanut oil), poultry, nuts, and seeds.
Omega-3 fatty acids	While no specific amount is recommended, the USDA guidelines advise eating foods rich in this healthy fat while staying within your total fat allowance.	Fatty cold-water fish (such as salmon, mackerel, and herring), ground flaxseed, flax oil, and walnuts.
Saturated fat	Limit saturated fat to no more than 10 percent of your total calories. Or to further reduce your heart disease risk, limit to 7 percent. Based on a 2,000-calorie-a-day diet, a 10 percent limit amounts to about 22 grams of saturated fat a day, while 7 percent is about 15 grams. Saturated fat intake counts toward your total daily allowance of fat.	Cheese, pizza, grain-based desserts, and animal products, such as chicken dishes, sausage, hot dogs, bacon, and ribs. Other sources: lard, butter, and coconut, palm, and other tropical oils.

Trans fat	USDA guidelines say the lower the better. Avoid trans fats from synthetic (processed) sources. It's difficult to eliminate all trans fats because they occur naturally in meat and dairy foods. The American Heart Association recommends limiting trans fat to no more than 1 percent of your total daily calories. For most people, this is less than 2 grams a day.	Margarines, snack foods, and prepared desserts, such as cookies and cakes. Naturally occurring sources include meat and dairy products.
Cholesterol	Less than 300 milligrams a day; less than 200 milligrams a day if you're at high risk of cardiovascular disease.	Eggs and egg dishes, chicken dishes, beef dishes, and hamburgers. Other sources: Seafood, dairy products, lard, and butter.

Source: Dietary Guidelines for Americans, 2010

FAT HABIT #32

*I just can't stand how I look right now. I want
to lose 10 pounds yesterday.* —AMBER B.

Your twenty-year reunion is just days away, and you'd love to lose 10 (or more) pounds before then. One word: impossible!

While there's no shortage of "crash" diets promising speedy weight loss, the reality is that there is no safe magic bullet to shrink your waistline overnight (or even over seven nights). You probably didn't gain the extra weight overnight, so it just isn't reasonable to expect to lose it in a few days. If you expect rapid weight loss, you are likely to be very disappointed.

Five Fast Fat Fixes

Adding more healthy fats and limiting unhealthy fats are a cinch with these five tips from the Harvard School for Public Health.

1. **Use liquid plant oils.** Olive, canola, and other plant-based oils are rich in heart-healthy unsaturated fats. Try dressing up a salad or roasted vegetables with an olive oil–based vinaigrette.

2. **Sleuth out trans fats.** In the supermarket, read the label to find foods that are trans fat–free. The label should say "0" (zero) on the line for trans fat. But before you toss it into your cart, you have to take one extra step: Scan the ingredient list to make sure it does not contain partially hydrogenated oils, because these oils are a source of trans fats and you want to avoid products containing them. According to government regulations, anything with fewer than 0.5 grams of trans fat can legally be called trans fat–free. Fortunately, most food manufacturers have removed trans fats from their products. In restaurants that don't have nutrition information readily available, steer clear of fried foods, biscuits, and other baked goods, unless you know that the restaurant has eliminated trans fats—many already have.

3. **Make the switch to soft tub margarine.** Choose a product that has zero grams of trans fat, and scan the ingredient list to make sure it does not contain partially hydrogenated oils. Even better, use a liquid plant oil whenever possible; refrigerated extra virgin olive oil makes a great spread for toast.

4. **Opt for omega-3 fats each day.** Have at least one serving daily of fatty fish (such as salmon and tuna), walnuts, or canola oil; all provide omega-3 fatty acids, essential fats.

5. **Cut back on red meat, cheese, milk, and ice cream.** Red meat (beef, pork, lamb) and full-fat dairy products are high in saturated fat. So eat less red meat (especially red processed meat, such as bacon), and choose fish, chicken, nuts, low-fat dairy, or beans instead. If/when you do eat red meat, choose lean cuts and stick to smaller portions.

SLIM SOLUTION

SKIP SHORTCUTS

The foundation of every successful weight-loss program remains a healthy, calorie-controlled diet combined with exercise. For successful, long-term weight loss, you must make permanent changes in your lifestyle and health habits. We, and most other experts, recommend aiming to lose 1 to 2 pounds (0.5 to 1 kilogram) a week.

"If you're eating and/or exercising in a way that you know you won't be able to maintain long-term, you're probably losing weight too fast and will likely gain some or all of it back. As you lose weight, you should feel energized and balanced, and your patterns should feel sustainable," says Cynthia Sass.

FAT HABIT #33

If I can't be superskinny it's not worth dieting. —JOAN G.

The average runway model stands about five-foot-ten and weighs in at 112 pounds—in most cases, setting a goal to look like her is both unrealistic and unhealthy. The most important factors that determine ideal weight are how you feel physically and emotionally, and how consistent you can be with your habits.

SLIM SOLUTION

BE FLEXIBLE

It's okay if you don't weigh what you weighed when you were 18. Many things change in your body over the years, and often people find they feel great and experience optimal health at a weight that's about 10 percent higher than the lowest weight from their college years.

Even if you can't get close to your lowest weight as an early adult, don't be discouraged. Research has shown that losing just 5 to 10 percent of your body weight can significantly lower your disease risk.

FAT HABIT #34

Diets are so rigid. They mean giving up my favorite foods. —JOHN C.

What's life without a little candy, some cookies, or a scoop of ice cream? The simple fact is that if you have to say no to your favorite foods all the time, it won't be too long before you snap, and start saying yes, yes, yes . . . to fettuccine Alfredo, French fries, margaritas, and oh, yes, chocolate!

SLIM SOLUTIONS

EMPHASIZE WHAT YOU *CAN* EAT

Healthy eating is all about learning to balance more indulgent, high-calorie foods with a wide selection of whole grains, fruits and veggies, lean protein, and healthy fats. (See Slim Solutions for Fat Habit #29, "I'm a yo-yo dieter.")

BE AN INTUITIVE EATER

This approach involves reconnecting with your feelings of hunger and satiety, or your body's "on/off hunger switch," so you can trust yourself with food and bring enjoyment back into eating. The underlying premise of intuitive eating is that you will learn to respond to your body. We were all born with the ability to eat intuitively, but our hunger and satiety cues are often clouded by years of dieting and misleading or downright incorrect food beliefs.

Interested in intuitive eating? Check out ten principles of intuitive eating, from RDs Evelyn Tribole and Elyse Resch, authors of *Intuitive Eating.*

INTUITIVE EATING PRINCIPLES

1. | *Reject the diet mentality.* Throw out the diet books and magazine articles that offer you false hope of losing weight quickly, easily, and permanently. Get angry at the lies that have led you to feel as if you were a failure every time a diet failed you. If you allow even one small hope to linger that a new and better diet might be lurking around the corner, it will prevent you from being free to rediscover intuitive eating.

2. | *Honor your hunger.* Feed your body with enough calories; otherwise you can trigger a primal drive to overeat. Once you reach the moment of excessive hunger, all intentions of moderate, conscious eating are easily forgotten. Learning to honor this first biological signal sets the stage for rebuilding trust with yourself and food.

3. | *Make peace with food.* Stop the food fight! Give yourself unconditional permission to eat. If you tell yourself that you can't or shouldn't have a particular food, it can lead to intense feelings of deprivation that build into uncontrollable cravings and, often, bingeing. When you finally "give in" to your forbidden food, eating will be experienced with such intensity, it usually results in overeating and overwhelming guilt.

4. | *Don't judge.* Put an end to those thoughts in your head that declare you're "good" for eating under 1,000 calories or "bad" because you ate a piece of chocolate cake. This food police mentality simply feeds into the unreasonable rules that dieting has created. Chasing the food police away is a critical step in returning to intuitive eating.

5. | *Respect your fullness.* Observe the signs that show that you're comfortably full, and use the Hunger Scale in Fat Habit #13. Pause in the middle of eating to ask yourself how the food tastes, and what your current fullness level is.

6. | *Discover the satisfaction factor.* Being healthy and enjoying food aren't mutually exclusive. The Japanese have the wisdom to prioritize pleasure, but in our quest to be thin, we often overlook one of the most basic gifts of existence: the joy and satisfaction that can be found in the eating experience. When you eat what you really want, in an environment that is inviting and positive, the pleasure you derive will be a powerful force that can help you feel satisfied and content. And you will probably find that it takes much less food for you to decide you've had "enough."

7. | *Divorce food from feelings.* Find ways to comfort, nurture, and distract yourself, or otherwise resolve your issues, without relying on food. Anxiety, loneliness, boredom, and anger are emotions we all experience throughout life—food won't fix any of them. It may comfort for the short term, distract from the pain, or even numb you into a food hangover. But in the long run, eating for emotional reasons will only make you feel worse. Sooner or later, you'll have to deal with the source of the emotion, and if you're an emotional eater, you'll have all those extra pounds to contend with too.

8. | *Respect your body.* Accept your genetic blueprint. Just as a person with a shoe size of eight would not expect to realistically squeeze into a size six, it is equally as futile (and uncomfortable) to have the same expectation with body size. But mostly, respect your body, so you can feel better about who you are. It's hard to reject the diet mentality if you are unrealistic and overly critical about your body shape.

9. | *Exercise—feel the difference.* Forget militant exercise that focuses solely on burning calories. Instead, pay attention to how it feels to move your body. If you think about how energized and confident you are after a workout, you'll be more likely to roll out of bed for a brisk morning walk. Believe it or not, calorie burning and weight loss are not the best motivators to skip the snooze button.

10. | *Create health with gentle nutrition.* Remember that you don't have to eat a perfect diet to be healthy. You will not suddenly get a nutrient deficiency or gain weight from a single snack, one meal, or a day of eating. It's what you eat consistently over time that matters—progress, not perfection, is what counts.

FAT HABIT #35

I have to eat perfectly to make a diet work. —JANE T.

There's no place for perfectionism in a healthy-eating plan. Strict all-or-nothing diets that are too restrictive and unrealistic are like trying to walk on a tightrope for life—eventually, nearly all of us fall off. Keep in mind, there is no such thing as perfect eating.

SLIM SOLUTION

Ban black-and-white thinking, abandon that all-or-nothing mentality, and forget about perfection. Instead, focus on strategies you can realistically live with. Also, realize that slipups happen to everyone—it's how you deal with a bad day, week, or month that helps predict success. Individuals who can lose weight and maintain that loss can be flexible enough with themselves to bounce back to healthy eating after a lapse.

Christen Cupples Cooper, MS, RD, founder of Cooper Nutrition Education & Communications (coopernutrition.com), offers the following strategies for getting back on track after you fall off the wagon:

- *Let go of guilt.* There is no sense in beating yourself up after overdoing it. The fact is, it takes approximately 3,500 calories above and beyond what your body uses in a day to equal a pound gained.
- *Avoid unnecessary extras.* "Extras" include things like creamy or oily salad dressing, alcoholic beverages, cookies, chips, or pretzels. It's the kind of stuff that you may enjoy, but you could easily live without.
- *No undereating.* Many people undereat the day after a big overindulgence. While this may seem like a good way to cut back on calories, it often just makes you so hungry that you're apt to overdo it again. Don't slam on the brakes and starve yourself.

FAT HABIT #36

I'm hooked on diet foods. —KAREN Z.

Remember when Snackwell's cookies first hit the scene? It was worse than a blowout sale at Bloomingdale's: Women went crazy for the no-fat and low-fat cookies, and grocery stores couldn't keep them in stock. There was only one problem: We wound up eating way more of these "diet-friendly" cookies than we would have eaten of the full-fat versions. (And let's be honest: The cookies didn't even taste that good!)

There are slimmed-down versions of just about every food you can imagine, but these diet aids are really diet hazards in disguise. Diet food that makes you fat—oh, the irony. Studies suggest that cutting calories by eating "diet" or low-calorie versions may actually produce a rebound effect. In other words, the more "diet" (low-calorie or even zero-calorie) sodas and foods you consume, the more you wind up eating.

There are a number of reasons this happens. On a psychological front, you may overeat a diet food, reasoning that it's not as bad as the full-fat or full-calorie version. (Just ask any woman who's ever polished off an entire box of "fat-free" cookies!) There's a physiological component as well; some research suggests that our bodies are preprogrammed to anticipate high-calorie fulfillment when drinking a soda or noshing on a sweet-tasting nibble. When our bodies don't receive those calories, we feel unsatisfied and end up eating more of something else to make up the difference. In other words, you may have temporarily tricked your brain into consuming fewer calories, but your body will probably compel you to offset the "savings" later on.

SLIM SOLUTIONS

INDULGE IN MODERATION

Remember that you can't eat unlimited quantities of *anything*, even a "light" version. Calories count, and even low-calorie products can add up quickly.

RETHINK "DIET" FOODS

Consider diet versions of foods a treat, and base your diet around whole grains, lean protein, fruits, and veggies. A healthful diet will help you feel satisfied without resorting to lightened-up versions of foods and beverages.

CUT THROUGH CONFUSING CLAIMS

Supermarkets are teeming with unhealthy "health" foods and beverages (see the box on the next page for a list of top offenders), which

Beware of Diet Deceivers

Be on the lookout for "healthy" foods that may not be so healthy after all, including:

- **Prepared "salads."** There's one basic diet fact that most people count on: salad = healthy. That's not necessarily true, especially when the salad you're selecting isn't even green. Already-prepared tuna salads, chicken salads, and shrimp salads are often loaded with fat and calories due to their high mayonnaise content. An overstuffed tuna sandwich can contain as many as 700 calories and 40 grams of fat! If you're ordering out, opt for prepared salads made with low-fat mayonnaise, and keep the portion to about the size of a deck of cards. Better yet, make your own, so you'll know exactly what's in it—and what's not.

- **Reduced-fat peanut butter.** A surprising news flash: Reduced-fat peanut butter isn't healthier than the regular version. Here's how they stack up: Both regular and reduced-fat peanut butter contain about the same number of calories; regular obviously has more fat, but it's the "good" monounsaturated fats that have made peanut butter a dieter's best friend. And reduced-fat versions have more sugar. Instead of choosing a lower-fat version, opt for a natural peanut butter with an ingredient list that contains no added sugar, or find a store where you can grind your own. And remember that peanut butter is high in calories, so watch your portions.

- **Smoothies.** Most smoothies start with a healthy enough foundation (low-fat dairy products and fruit), but when you add sugar, ice cream, or sherbet, they go from healthy to horrendous. Plus, their serving sizes are huge (the smallest is often 16 ounces). It's all too easy to slurp down 500 calories in one glass. Gulp! While a smoothie can be a great way to start the day or refuel post-workout, you have to account for those calories.

- **Flavored yogurt.** Flavored yogurt has double the sugar content of plain, which means you're adding four extra teaspoons to a healthy snack. Not so sweet! A better bet: Choose plain, low-fat, or no-fat yogurt and stir in a teaspoon of honey, maple syrup, or all-fruit spread for a hint of sweetness. Or go Greek: Fat-free Greek yogurt, which is lower in sugar than even regular plain yogurt but often contains twice as much protein, will keep you satisfied longer.

- **Granola/energy bars.** Granola or energy bars are the perfect pre-workout or between-meal snack, right? Not always. Many bars are loaded with high-fructose corn syrup, added sugar, and artery-clogging saturated fat. Plus, some bars (particularly meal-replacement varieties) contain more than 350 calories each—that's a lot more than a "snack" for most of us.

are marketed to make you think they're diet-friendly. They may have labels that read "Made with Whole Grains!" or "Fat-free" or "All Natural," but that doesn't mean they're a smart choice. When shopping for foods, make sure you understand what these common labels actually mean:

- *Fat-free.* Fat-free doesn't mean *calorie*-free! And just because a food is free of fat doesn't mean it's a health food. (Think gummy bears.) Of course, there are many healthy fat-free foods (most fruits and vegetables fit the bill!), but they're *naturally* fat-free. Read the nutrition labels when buying packaged foods to be sure you're getting something that's actually good for you—check calories, sodium, fiber, and vitamins and minerals—not just a food that's "fat-free."
- *Sugar-free.* Most foods labeled as "sugar-free"—like soda, candy, and other treats—are unhealthy foods to begin with. To make a product sugar-free, manufacturers replace traditional sweeteners with blends of natural or synthetic sugar substitutes. Research is

Your Guide to Decoding Food Labels

When it comes to eating healthfully, the eyes have it! When you use your peepers to read product labels, you can easily suss out the good-for-you foods from the not-so-good. Unfortunately, most Americans read "Nutrition Facts" (that's the formal name for where you can find a food's specs) about as often as they read the fine print on their credit card bills. And experts (including us) believe the reason people don't read labels is because they're too confusing and it's hard to easily translate them into information we can actually use.

Let's face it: Most people (who don't have a degree in nutrition) don't know a DV ("daily value") from the DMV. That's why the Centers for Disease Control, the Food and Drug Administration, and the Institute of Medicine are currently working to create a more user-friendly standard food label. At the same time, the food industry is creating its own strategies for marketing "nutrition" on their food packages (with claims like "contains whole grains" or "low-fat," as we mentioned earlier). There's always a battle going on, and you're the prime defender of your health.

To help simplify the Nutrition Facts panel and food labels in general, we polled fellow dietitians about the most important piece of information on a food label. Here are their top five recommendations of what to look for before buying any food, in order of importance:

1. **Serving size.** Without looking at what a "serving" is, everything else on the label is irrelevant. Yet this is one thing many of us overlook—until we realize that the package contained three servings, not one. Oops!
2. **Servings per package.** Many packaged foods may appear to contain one serving when they actually contain two or more. (This is one of the FDA's pet peeves about the current food labels.) This piece of info tells you how many servings you'd end up consuming if you ate the whole package. Having **"servings per package"** and **"calories per package"** in bold lettering on the front of a food package would help solve this issue, but in the meantime, make sure you check the label.

3. **Calories.** Virtually everyone should be aware of how many calories they consume, so check the calorie count of a product before buying. As a general rule, expect to consume about 450 to 650 calories for a meal and less than 200 for a snack.

4. **Saturated fat.** Choose foods that contain little saturated fat; most women should limit their intake to no more than 15 to 17 grams of saturated fat per day. The number one source of saturated fat in the U.S. diet is full-fat cheese (followed by pizza), so watch your portions of these potentially problematic foods.

5. **Sodium.** The less processed a food is, the lower its sodium content will be. Simply watching your sodium intake will automatically improve your diet, as you'll be choosing less-processed foods in favor of ones that are naturally sodium-free.

still unclear about whether using sugar substitutes will help you lose weight. Many experts believe (and we agree!) that artificial sweeteners intensify your desire for sweet foods—and make you less likely to be satisfied with the natural sweetness of an apple, banana, or papaya.

• *"Contains whole grains."* This claim is popping up on all kinds of chips, crackers, cookies, and breads. All a manufacturer has to do is add some form of whole grain to their food and they can slap a "Made with whole grain" or "Contains whole grains" claim on the label. The benefits of whole grains, like brown rice, oats, quinoa, and barley, have been well established. They can help reduce the risk of developing heart disease and certain cancers, and they're linked with lower overall body weight, possibly because of their high fiber content. But simply adding some whole grains to a cracker, cookie, cereal bar, or even a doughnut doesn't make it a healthy choice.

- *"Natural" and "all-natural" foods.* "Natural" means next to nothing on a food package. In fact, you can find "all-natural" claims on foods that contain high-fructose corn syrup, genetically modified ingredients, thickeners and stabilizers, and all kinds of other ingredients that aren't at all natural! According to the FDA, foods can sport the "natural" label as long as they don't contain synthetic additives, flavorings, or coloring agents. Bottom line: Don't be fooled by "natural" claims.

FAT HABIT #37

I'm on a gluten-free diet. —ZOE J.

Just over three million Americans—about one in a hundred—has celiac disease, a hereditary autoimmune disorder that causes the immune system to attack the small intestines when gluten, a protein found in many grains (for more details on gluten, check out the sidebar on the next page), is consumed. Research estimates that an additional eighteen million Americans have nonceliac gluten sensitivity, a condition in which a person cannot tolerate gluten and experiences symptoms similar to those with celiac disease but lacks the antibodies and intestinal damage seen in celiac disease.

Some sixty million Americans buy gluten-free foods—even though the vast majority of them are actually gluten-tolerant. Many choose this type of diet because they hope it will help them lose weight or cut back on the foods they eat too much of—breads, pasta, crackers, and baked goods.

But in some cases, avoiding gluten can actually make you *gain* weight. Here's why: The majority of processed gluten-free foods available at supermarkets tend to be crackers, cookies, desserts, and

What Is Gluten, Anyway?

Gluten is a protein found in wheat, barley, and rye (oats do not contain gluten naturally, but they're often processed in facilities that handle wheat or other gluten-containing grains). Gluten gives elasticity to dough, helping it rise and keep its shape, and often contributes a chewy texture to the final product. Gluten is also used as a stabilizing agent in foods like ketchup, ice cream, marinades, and salad dressings. It's a common additive and is often used in sauces, seasonings, soups, cold cuts, hot dogs, snack chips, and dietary supplements

other "treat"-type foods that we should be trying to limit. A gluten-free cookie is still made with sugars and fat, and while the flour it contains may be different, the calories rarely are.

In fact, gluten-free foods may be higher in calories than their gluten-containing counterparts. An afternoon at a local supermarket revealed that many gluten-free versions of pasta, muffins, and bread were considerably lower in fiber and nutrients, and higher in starchy calories as well as sugar and fat, compared to food with gluten, and especially compared to whole-grain products. For instance, one whole-grain English muffin had 120 calories, 1 gram of fat, and 3 grams of fiber per serving; the gluten-free version had 200 calories, a whopping 5 grams of fat, and 2 grams of fiber. A whole-wheat pasta brand had 120 calories, 1 gram of fat, and 3 grams of fiber; the gluten-free variety: 190 calories, 1 gram of fat, and 2 grams of fiber.

SLIM SOLUTION

MAKE A DATE WITH YOUR DOC

If you suspect you have celiac disease or nonceliac gluten sensitivity, it's important that you see your doctor. Accurately diagnosing these conditions can be quite difficult, largely because the symptoms often mimic those of other diseases, including irritable bowel syndrome (IBS), Crohn's disease, intestinal infections, lactose intolerance, and depression.

Blood tests are the first step in diagnosing celiac disease. A doctor will order one or more of a series of blood tests to measure your body's response to gluten.

It's important to continue eating a normal, gluten-containing diet before being tested for celiac. If the blood tests and symptoms indicate celiac, a physician may suggest a biopsy of the lining of the small intestine to confirm the diagnosis.

Don't give up on gluten if you can eat it. There's no reason to go "gluten-free" if you are gluten tolerant.

FAT HABIT #38

I have no clue what a "portion" looks like.
I just load up my plate.

—SUZANNE L.

Bigger isn't always better—especially when it comes to serving sizes. The statistics are startling: Twenty years ago, a typical cheeseburger had 330 calories; today it's closer to 600 calories. A side of French fries twenty years ago were a 2.4-ounce handful totaling 210 calories; today the standard order is a heaping 6.9 ounces, packing 610 calories. Remember 4-ounce juice glasses and wineglasses, or

---

Serving Size Shocker

7-Eleven stores sold 12- and 20-ounce sodas in the 1970s. By 1988, they were selling a 64-ounce "Double Gulp." That's a half gallon of soda being marketed for individual consumption!

8-ounce bottles of soda? No? Well, at one time they were standard sizes. Now they look like shot glasses!

It's no coincidence that as portions have grown, so have waistlines. In the 1960s, less than 15 percent of Americans were obese. Today that number is more than 40 percent.

Why are pumped-up portions such a problem? Studies show that the more food put in front of you, the more you eat. Our brains are programmed to eat with our eyes and not our stomachs, so when we're served a larger portion, we'll generally eat the whole thing, even if it makes us uncomfortably full.

And worse, many people don't even realize that what looks like a "normal" portion is actually a supersize serving. Restaurant chains are among the biggest offenders, and Americans spend nearly half of their food budget on foods prepared outside of the home. They consume about one-third of their daily calories from outside sources, much of it from fast food.

SLIM SOLUTIONS

There's no way around it: If you want to get a handle on your weight, you have to get smart about serving sizes. But there is a perk to paring down your portions: You can do it without feeling hungry. One study in the *American Journal of Clinical Nutrition* found that women who shrank their portions by 25 percent slashed 250 calories a day—enough to help them lose a half pound a week while still feeling full.

Go from supersize to "smart size" using these strategies:

PUT PORTIONS IN PERSPECTIVE

Your first step to becoming a portion pro is getting familiar with what a healthy portion looks like. Use the list of common foods and single-serving equivalents below to get some portion perspective.

What Does One Serving Look Like?

GRAIN PRODUCTS

1 cup of cereal flakes = a fist

1 pancake = a compact disc

½ cup of cooked rice, pasta, or potato = ½ baseball

1 slice of bread = a CD case

1 piece of corn bread = a bar of soap

VEGETABLES AND FRUIT

1 cup of salad greens = a baseball

1 baked potato = a fist

1 medium fruit = a baseball

½ cup of fresh fruit = ½ baseball

¼ cup of raisins = a large egg

DAIRY AND CHEESE

1½ ounces of cheese = 4 stacked dice or 2 cheese slices

½ cup of ice cream = ½ baseball

1 teaspoon margarine or spread = 1 die

Serving Size Card

1 SERVING LOOKS LIKE . . .

Grain Products

1 cup of cereal flakes = fist

1 pancake = compact disc

½ cup of cooked rice, pasta,
   or potato = ½ baseball

1 slice of bread = CD case

1 piece of corn bread = bar of soap

1 SERVING LOOKS LIKE . . .

Vegetables and Fruit

1 cup of salad greens = baseball

1 baked potato = fist

1 medium fruit = baseball

½ cup of fresh fruit = ½ baseball

¼ cup of raisins = large egg

1 SERVING LOOKS LIKE . . .

Dairy and Cheese

1½ oz. cheese = 4 stacked dice
   or 2 cheese slices

½ cup of ice cream = ½ baseball

1 tsp. margarine or spreads = 1 dice

1 SERVING LOOKS LIKE . . .

Meat and Alternatives

3 oz. meat, fish, or poultry =
   deck of cards

3 oz. grilled/baked fish = checkbook

2 Tbsp. peanut butter = Ping-Pong ball

MEAT AND ALTERNATIVES

3 ounces meat, fish, or poultry = a deck of cards

3 ounces grilled or baked fish = a checkbook

2 tablespoons of peanut butter = a Ping-Pong ball

DIVIDE AND CONQUER

Here's a simple rule to portion your plate properly: Divide it in half, and automatically fill one side with fruits or vegetables, leaving the rest for equal parts protein and starch. This way, you begin to see what a properly balanced meal looks like. Spaghetti and meatballs? Steak and potatoes? They're only half a meal—incomplete without fruits and vegetables.

UNPLUG

The TV, computer, and other electronic gadgets distract you from how much you're eating. The more you tune in to the tube or stare at the screen, the more food you're likely to stuff down your throat. In a study comparing how much popcorn viewers ate during a half-hour versus an hour-long show, those who watched more television ate 28 percent more popcorn. For more on putting down that remote, see Fat Habit #56, "I get sucked into the TV."

SET A SKINNY TABLE

Did you know that the way you set your table can influence how many calories you eat? There are some simple ways you can change your home environment to reduce your calorie intake. For instance, research shows that going from a 12-inch plate to a 10-inch plate can reduce how much you eat by about 22 percent. And don't worry—you won't go hungry; using a smaller plate fools your brain into thinking you are satisfied on fewer calories!

The same is true for smaller bowls and spoons. Smaller serving spoons were found to result in a 14 percent decrease in food intake, while smaller bowls led to a whopping 50 percent decrease in eating. For more on setting your table for weight-loss success, see Fat Habit #57 "I like to fill up my plate—and my dishes are huge!" and Fat Habit #63, "We serve our meals family-style."

FORGET FAMILY-STYLE

Leave giant platters of food on the table and what's going to happen? People will eat it. That may seem obvious, but so many of us put extra food out on the table, making second and third helpings much more likely. After you've plated everyone's food, leave pots, pans, and platters on the counter or stove—you're less likely to go back for more if you have to get up for it.

DINING OUT? DOGGIE-BAG IT!

Some of the biggest portion pitfalls happen when dining out. Restaurants supersize everything from salads to sundaes. As soon as you get your entrée, doggie-bag half of it even before you start eating.

Other ways to cut calories when you're out and about:

- Ask about half portions or appetizer-size plates, or order from the children's menu.
- Share an entrée with your companion.
- Eat a healthy appetizer and soup or salad instead of an entrée.

For more on how to dine out without overdoing it, see Chapter 6.

FAT HABIT #39

I'm a vegetarian—as long as I don't eat meat or dairy,
I'll be healthy and lean. —JESSIE S.

There's no doubt that a vegetarian diet, one that includes no meat or fish, can be one of the healthiest ways to eat. Studies show that vegetarians tend to have lower rates of obesity, heart disease, and high blood pressure. But there's a lot of variation with vegetarianism. For instance, for some people, "vegetarianism means a diet of Cheez Doodles, nonfat frozen yogurt, a few pieces of fruit, and maybe a cookie or two," says Katherine.

In other words, being a vegetarian does *not* guarantee you good health or a healthy weight if your calories are coming from the wrong foods. Whether you're a vegan (someone who avoids all animal products, including meat, dairy, and eggs) or someone who just won't eat meat or poultry, it's important that your version of vegetarianism still controls for calories and chooses the healthiest picks so you get all the nutrients you need.

SLIM SOLUTIONS

COUNT CALORIES

Even if you're eliminating animal products from your diet, you can still go awry if you compensate by overeating high-fat, high-calorie foods. Keep track of calories to make sure you're not overdoing it.

GO FOR VARIETY

Ensure that you're eating a well-balanced diet by including a variety of fruits, veggies, nuts, seeds, legumes, and whole grains. If you are less strict about your vegetarianism, also consider incorporating dairy and eggs in your diet to add protein.

COVER YOUR NUTRITIONAL BASES

Vegetarians and especially vegans can easily fall short on protein, vitamin B12, iron, zinc, calcium, and vitamin D. Be sure you are choosing foods higher in these nutrients, or speak with your physician about taking supplements.

DO YOUR HOMEWORK

If you're thinking of becoming a vegetarian, we suggest doing some research first, or working with a registered dietitian with experience in vegetarian diets. Check out some of the resources below:

The Academy of Nutrition and Dietetics—www.eatright.org

The American Heart Association—www.americanheart.org

ChooseMyPlate tips for vegetarians—www.choosemyplate.gov/
healthy-eating-tips/tips-for-vegetarian.html

International Vegetarian Union—www.ivu.org

The Vegetarian Resource Group—www.vrg.org

VegSource—www.vegsource.com

A "detox" diet is the only way to lose belly fat.

—FRANCISCA W.

Detox diets may have a huge following among celebrities (Gwyneth Paltrow and Beyoncé have reportedly used them to get red-carpet ready), but they're not so popular among dietitians. "I recently went to a food show where several 'cleanse and detox' diets were featured. I don't know what bothered me more: that people make tons of money with bogus detox claims or that so many consumers actually believe the hype," Katherine says.

Of course, it's not just celebrities who are dabbling in detox diets. We get questions all the time from clients about the potential benefits of "detoxing," "cleansing," and fasting. With the rise in popularity of BluePrintCleanse and similar plans, we're hearing about more and more people who turn to so-called detoxification programs to lose weight, shed belly fat, clear up acne, and even increase fertility. But before you forsake your fork, you should know the skinny on cleansing, fasting, and detoxing, including what each is and whether it offers any benefits.

FASTING AND WEIGHT LOSS

Most medical experts and RDs do *not* recommend fasting as a way to lose weight. Although a drastic cut in calories may seem like the speediest way to slim down, this approach can backfire. When you go back to your usual diet, your lowered metabolism doesn't get the memo to speed back up. The result: You may store more energy, so you'll likely gain back the weight you lost—and possibly even put on *more* weight, even though you're eating the same number of calories as you did before your fast.

FASTING TO "DETOXIFY" THE BODY

Many fad diets include a "detox" phase, during which dieters are instructed to drink only water, juice, or herbal teas. But there is scant scientific evidence showing that fasting will detox or cleanse your body. Fasting does *not* boost the body's disposal system.

SLIM SOLUTIONS

INVEST YOUR MONEY ELSEWHERE

Save what you would have spent on detox formulas and juices, and use it instead on a gym membership, new sneakers, or fitness gear. That's money well spent.

CHECK IN WITH YOUR DOCTOR

For most healthy individuals, a short-term fast isn't harmful. That said, if you are considering any type of fast, it is *imperative* that you check with your doctor first. Fasting can be dangerous for some people, including pregnant and breast-feeding women, the elderly, and individuals with certain health conditions.

CLEANSE YOUR BODY THE HEALTHY WAY

Eating a sensible diet with plenty of fruits, vegetables, whole grains, lean protein, and unsaturated fats will keep your body running efficiently. (See our sample meal plan in Chapter 7 for more details.)

FAT HABIT #41

I diet by skipping meals. Fewer meals mean fewer calories.

—AMBER T.

It seems like basic math: Cut calories by cutting a meal here and there, and you'll lose weight. Except that's not how it works. This common diet trick backfires on almost everyone who tries it. People who skip meals—especially breakfast—consume more total calories during the day compared with those who do not. Why? Meal skippers tend to snack more, and eat larger meals and higher-calorie foods.

Breakfast may seem like the easiest meal to skip—most people would rather score an extra ten minutes of slumber than whip up a healthy morning meal. Refuse the siren song of the snooze button! Breakfast helps jump-start metabolism and sets the stage for managing hunger throughout the day.

SLIM SOLUTIONS

EAT THREE SQUARES

The most recent weight-loss research recommends a "normalized" eating pattern of three squares and a midmorning and midafternoon snack.

BREAK FOR BREAKFAST

Start your day with a wholesome, filling breakfast of about 300 to 400 calories and at least 20 grams of satisfying protein. Check out three of Julie's favorite breakfasts:

* A bowl of oatmeal (1 cup cooked) with fresh fruit and ¼ cup of nonfat plain Greek yogurt

- 1 whole egg and 1 to 2 egg whites (or 4 egg whites) with roasted veggies with 1 slice of whole-wheat toast
- A container of low-fat or nonfat Greek yogurt with fresh fruit mixed with ¼ cup oats or Grape-Nuts

For more great meal ideas, follow our meal plan in Chapter 7.

FAT HABIT #42

I believe in magic bullets! —JOANNE C.

Americans plunk down $40 billion each year on diet products. Most of the quick-fix weight-loss industry—replete with phony pills such as raspberry ketones, powders, and potions, like the hCG diet, that claim to melt away pounds with little or no effort—can be summed up in one word: bogus.

There are dozens of weight-loss scams out there. Some of the worst offenders include:

- ***The Pure Energy weight-loss band.*** This plastic bracelet is embedded with green and silver hologram disks claimed to give off vibes that resonate throughout the body and stimulate weight loss and health. Among the promised results are decreased appetite, balanced metabolism, balanced hormones, enhanced energy flow, increased energy levels, and the promotion of positive emotions.
- ***Sensa weight-loss crystals.*** The Sensa website states boldly that users can lose an average of 30.5 pounds in six months without dieting, exercise, food restrictions, or drastic lifestyle changes. All you have to do: Sprinkle weight-loss crystals on your food.

Class-action suits have been filed against the marketers of Sensa, stating that (A) there is no competent and reliable scientific evidence to substantiate these claims, and (B) an expert who reviewed Sensa's main clinical study judged it "beyond worthless."

- *The hCG (human chorionic gonadotropin) diet.* HCG was first introduced more than fifty years ago by British physician Albert Simeon, who claimed the hormone, found in the urine of pregnant women, would mobilize stored fat, suppress appetite, and redistribute fat. He contended that regular injections would enable dieters to live comfortably on a 500-calorie-a-day diet. Anyone taking in 500 calories would lose weight quickly—but the "comfortably" claim? Studies haven't found any evidence of this. Despite the celebrity testimonials and widespread marketing, hCG is not effective or legal, and may be harmful.

Drops, shots, pills, powders, and potions will lighten up one thing: your wallet. Short of bariatric surgery, there are currently no products that are proven effective for long-term weight loss. What works: a healthy, calorie-controlled diet and a regular exercise program.

SLIM SOLUTIONS

BE PATIENT
If you want to lose weight the healthy way—so it stays off—you have to accept that it takes time and commitment.

DON'T BE DUPED
As we said at the beginning of this chapter, if it sounds too good to be true, it probably is.

LOOK NO FARTHER THAN YOUR SUPERMARKET FOR A WEIGHT-LOSS SOLUTION THAT WORKS

The best diet foods are readily available and won't drain your wallet: Eat a diet rich in plant-based foods like whole grains, fruits, and vegetables. They're the most nutrient-rich and filling. Follow the weight-loss advice in this book, and not only will you be slimmer, you'll be healthier too!

I'M CLUELESS WHEN IT COMES TO SHOPPING AND COOKING

ARE YOU ON A FIRST-NAME BASIS WITH THE PIZZA DELIVERY GUY? Do you know the local taqueria shop's number by heart? Do you get lost in the supermarket? Or worse, have you never actually shopped at your supermarket?

If you answered yes to any of these questions, then you're part of the growing majority of Americans who'd rather make dinner reservations than dinner. More than eight in ten adults eat out once a week, while more than half dine out two or more times per week. Away-from-home meals have skyrocketed since the 1970s—along with the nation's waistline.

Eating out makes it harder to manage your weight, no matter how disciplined you are. It's time to show your stove some love; doing so allows you to control ingredients, calories, and ultimately your weight. In this chapter, you'll find loads of strategies to help you feel more at home in your own kitchen.

FAT HABIT #43

Living in San Francisco, I eat almost all my meals out because we
have the best restaurants. Even the street food is better
than anything I can make. —HEATHER B.

We feel your pain on this one. Both of us have lived in food lovers' cities for a time: Katherine is a native New Yorker, and Julie also lived there for eighteen years before moving just minutes from San Francisco. But the truth is, you don't have to reside in a major city to be tempted by restaurant fare. Whether you live in San Francisco or Shreveport, Des Moines or Decatur, you're sure to have endless options for ethnic cuisine, cafés, Michelin-rated restaurants, food trucks, delis, or diners. And if you frequent any of these places, you'll likely exceed your daily calories.

Study after study shows that dining out and weight gain go hand in hand. One study published in the *Journal of the American Dietetic Association* found that women who ate out most frequently consumed nearly **300 more calories a day** compared with women who ate out once or twice weekly. An extra 300 calories a day could equal more than 20 pounds in a year!

Part of the problem is that we think more about our wallets than our waists: Too many of us try to get our money's worth when we eat out. Another hazard: Healthy-sounding options are often far from healthy.

Consider the average calorie count of restaurant dishes from a national survey of U.S. restaurants:

Appetizers: 813 calories
Main entrées: 675 calories
Salads: 500 calories

Salad dressings: 175 calories

Side dishes: 260 calories

Soups: 225 calories

Specialty nonalcoholic beverages: 420 calories

Even if you ordered just a soup and salad (with dressing), you'd be scarfing down 900 calories! That one "light meal" is equivalent to two meals on our meal plans and is 56 percent of your total daily calories. Doesn't sound so light now, does it? No matter which combo you choose, it adds up to weight gain.

SLIM SOLUTION

The only way to keep a lid on calories (as well as fat, sugar, and sodium) is to take food prep into your own hands. Work on gradually cutting back on the number of meals you order out or eat out until you get down to our recommendation of no more than two meals eaten out per week. Keep on reading—you'll find more great tips and tricks in this chapter to help make it a smooth transition.

FAT HABIT #44

Healthy recipes are too much work and require special ingredients.

—VALERIE B.

Actually, we've found it's just the opposite. Unhealthy recipes often require more: more ingredients, more sauces, more gravies, more toppings—more effort. Some of the healthiest dishes we've come across call for less than a handful of ingredients. For instance, you can whip up a healthy chicken dish using only chicken, lemon, salt, and pepper. Doesn't get much easier than that!

The key to creating nutritious meals and snacks is using wholesome foods like fresh fruits and vegetables, whole grains, fresh lean protein, and healthy fats. Consider some other healthy dishes you can pull together in a hurry: grilled poultry, beef, or seafood; salads with lean protein; roasted chicken and vegetables; pastas and pizza. None of these are hard to make, and no special ingredients are required.

Let's face it: Recipes that feature lengthy lists of ingredients or foods you can't even pronounce are intimidating—even for the most seasoned chef. If this is your problem, then you've come to the right place. Our cooking MO is to ensure that everything we make calls for only a few ingredients and doesn't require too much of our most precious commodity—time.

SLIM SOLUTION

Check out the recipes in Chapter 9; you'll be surprised by how simple and speedy it can be to cook like a nutrition pro. In fact, most of our recipes require fewer than eight readily available ingredients and take less than thirty minutes to prepare. The most you'll need to do is boil, bake, grill, or roast. That's it. Sounds appetizing, right?

FAT HABIT #45

Healthy recipes never taste good. —NINA S.

For some reason, delicious and healthy have become mutually exclusive. Most people are under the mistaken impression that you can't have both; it's either good flavor or good health. In fact, studies show that when food companies use a healthy descriptor on a product, people assume it won't taste as good.

We say, why choose? That's right—you *can* have both! There is a growing movement among many chefs and chefs-in-training to cook lighter dishes; they're dropping fattening meats and fried foods with heavy sauces from their menus and serving more fantastic dishes that put veggies, fruit, and lean meats forward. One taste of our recipes (flip to Chapter 9 for our best recipes) and you'll see exactly what we mean. And feel free to use the following tricks to create your own healthy and (yes!) tasty recipes.

SLIM SOLUTIONS

USE FRESH INGREDIENTS

Have you ever picked a tomato and eaten it off the vine? Blueberries straight from the bush? If so, you know how flavorful and delicious fresh foods taste. They're so good on their own, they don't need anything to dress them up. We know it's not always possible to use fresh, but using more fresh, in-season ingredients like vegetables, fruits, and herbs from farmers' markets can help you taste the difference of fresh food.

BE SPICY

Use more fresh and dried herbs and spices—nothing adds more calorie-free flavor to foods. An added bonus: Some herbs and spices will actually add a modest boost to your metabolism.

DRESS IT UP

Quick and easy vinaigrettes (like Julie's recipe below) are an easy way to make cooked veggies or salad greens taste even better. There are thousands of variations on vinaigrette, so try different ones on for size.

JULIE'S FAVORITE VINAIGRETTE

⅓ cup extra virgin olive oil
¼ cup champagne vinegar
2 teaspoons shallots, minced
2 teaspoons stone-ground mustard
Salt and pepper to taste

■ Put all ingredients in a sealable jar and shake vigorously. Store in an airtight container in the refrigerator for up to a week. Return to room temperature before using.

GO NUTS

Toasting brings out the flavor of nuts and other foods, so you can use a little less in recipes. Toasted almonds, pine nuts, walnuts, pistachios, or pecans can add great taste and texture to meals and snacks.

SAY CHEESE!

A little cheese can turn a dish from blah to ahh! We use a lot of feta cheese, goat cheese, and Parmesan. A helpful hint: When you shred cheese, you get more volume and it disperses into your dishes, making them taste richer without adding much extra fat or calories.

FAKE IT

Who doesn't love the taste of fried food? What we don't love: all those extra calories! Our compromise: "mock" fried foods, like faux crispy fried chicken tenders, oven-baked crispy fried fish, sweet potato fries, zucchini fries, and other amazing dishes that have all the flavor—without all the fat—of fried foods.

FAT HABIT #46

I feel lost in my supermarket . . . there are just so many choices.

—NANCY M.

Supersize supermarkets are packing in more products than ever. Take a look at these numbers (and be prepared to hold on to your cart): In the 1970s, grocery stores stocked about 7,000 products. Today the average store carries about 40,000 different products, with some of the larger stores packing in 50,000 different items. And, of course, most of these new foods are processed— as opposed to fruits and veggies and other healthy perishables. In fact, the percentage of diet-friendly items is shrinking in relation to high-calorie, high-fat, high-sugar processed products.

The reason for the increased offerings is simple: It increases sales. The more variety in the store, the more we buy. And, of course, the more we buy, the more we eat, and ultimately the harder it is to button up those jeans.

Unless you're lucky enough to live near a smaller, family-owned food store with more limited offerings, you're stuck with these ginormous grocery stores. Fortunately, if you know how to navigate your cart through the aisles and are aware of common—and very effective—marketing tricks, you can get out with your diet still intact. Our GPS guide below will help you survive the supermarket.

SLIM SOLUTIONS

MAKE A LIST

Don't even think about setting foot in the store without one! If you do, you risk being influenced by food manufacturers' and retailers' advertising, promotions, and in-store marketing tools designed to get you to buy more. To create skinny shopping lists, see Fat Habit #51, "I never use a shopping list."

READ SIGNS

Those signs hanging from the ceiling telling you which products are down which aisles can be a huge help. Read them—and then steer clear of the aisles that contain foods you don't want to bring home, like snack foods, crackers, candy, soda, and baked goods.

RELY ON LABELS

You may have heard that you should stick to the perimeter of the store, because that's typically where the healthiest foods are found. That's not always true—they may be scattered throughout the store. The only surefire way to sleuth out the best products is to read labels. "Smart shoppers know that reading labels is how to determine whether a food is healthy, not by the location of the item," explains Leah McGrath, RD, LDN, the corporate dietitian for Ingles Markets.

LOOK HIGH AND LOW

The least healthy and most expensive foods are usually placed at or slightly below eye level on store shelves. Look higher and lower within categories to find the more nutritious options.

BYPASS THE BAKERY

The aroma of just-baked breads, cookies, and cakes is a real test of anyone's willpower. The best way to cope is to stay as far away from the bakery counter as possible.

SKIP SAMPLES

Most supermarkets entice us with samples of baked goods, cheese, snack foods, and much more. Politely decline these sampling opportunities, because you may feel obligated to buy.

Shopping by the Numbers

- Two-thirds of buying decisions are made in-store, making shoppers more susceptible to marketing.
- In a typical shopping trip, shoppers spend 60 to 80 percent of their time pushing their carts up and down aisles aimlessly. Those who meander the most spend up to twice as much at the checkout counter.
- Shoppers read only eight to ten lines of copy in a shopping trip and purchase based on flashy in-store displays and packaging color. Icons influence most purchases.
- Foods that are positioned at the end of aisles and face three directions account for 30 to 40 percent of all supermarket sales.

AVOID END-OF-AISLE PURCHASES

End-of-aisle displays, which usually feature less nutritious options, are very eye-catching. Don't be influenced to purchase items in these spots.

CHECK FOR HEALTHY SYMBOLS

Many supermarkets use icons or other nutritional guidance systems to help you spot the healthier choices. For example, Whole Foods stores use the ANDI system, others use a system called NuVal, and some chains have their own proprietary system. Ask your store manager whether your supermarket has a better-for-you shopping system. Studies show that these programs help to shift purchases to more nutritious choices.

FINISH WITH FROZEN

For food safety reasons, you want to minimize the amount of time perishables are without refrigeration. To keep your perishables and frozen foods safe, pick up your nonperishables first; then shop for refrigerated and frozen items.

DON'T DAWDLE

Pushing your cart up and down each aisle just creates more opportunities to toss something you don't want or need into your cart. Head straight to the checkout when you've gotten everything on your list.

FAT HABIT #47

I don't know what I should be looking at on the food labels to tell whether a product is good for me. —KIM K.

Reading a food label seems about as exciting as reading the manual to your smartphone. It's not just the snooze factor—reading labels takes time.

The truth is, if you want to lose weight and keep it off, you have to learn to love labels. Research shows that shoppers who regularly read nutrition labels and comparison-shop for products are less likely to be overweight, and have better diets than those who avoid reading labels.

SLIM SOLUTIONS

The key to using the food label to your advantage is to know what to pay attention to and what you can ignore. Yes—skipping parts is allowed! Here's what you can ignore:

HEALTH AND NUTRITION CLAIMS

"Big claims on the front of a package are often a clue that the product doesn't measure up nutritionally," says Susan Moores, MS, RD, the nutritionist for Kowalski's Markets in the Twin Cities. Front-of-pack statements like "all-natural," "low-fat," "sugar-free," and "reduced in sodium" mean little when it comes to your health, so don't assume products with these claims should be in your shopping cart.

In addition, "organic" doesn't always mean "diet-friendly." Organic refers to the way an item was produced (meeting the USDA organic standards) and has nothing to do with how nutritious it is. For instance, organic brownies or cookies won't get your scale going in the right direction.

Another trap many dieters fall for: "gluten-free." It may seem like a product sporting this label is better for you, but many of the gluten-free options are loaded with naturally gluten-free ingredients, like sugar, fat, sodium, and calories! (See Fat Habit #37, "I'm on a gluten-free diet.")

Turn the package over to the back or side to find the Nutrition Facts, and focus on the three items below to determine which foods are calorie bombs and which are calorie bargains.

SERVING SIZE AND SERVINGS PER PACKAGE

Serving size will be the first item on the Nutrition Facts panel, and next to it you'll find the total number of servings in a package. This is important—the frozen pizza you bought may say one slice is a serving, but the package contains eight servings. If you split this equally with someone, you're each eating four servings. It can be confusing, because many people make the mistake of thinking one product equals one serving, but that's not always the case.

CALORIES PER SERVING

When you look at the serving size and calories per serving, you can immediately figure out whether this food fits into your calorie budget. Remember, our meal plans are set for 1,600 calories or 1,800 calories for women to promote weight loss. Those calories, divided among your meals and snacks, would look like this:

WOMEN: 1,600 CALORIES
- Breakfast: 400 calories
- Snack: up to 200 calories
- Lunch: 400 calories
- Snack: up to 200 calories
- Dinner: 400 calories

For 1,800 calories, add another 200-calorie snack, or increase calories of any meal by 200.

If you pick up a bag of chips and read that one serving has 350 calories in it, you might want to put it back (unless that's about all you plan to eat for lunch). On the other hand, you may pick up a package of whole-grain flat breads and be shocked to find it has a reasonable serving size and less than 100 calories per serving. (Refer to Chapter 9 and guidelines.)

You want a food that will quash cravings, not create them, so limiting foods with added sugars to less than **100 calories, or 25 grams of added sugars per day** will help.

On the food label, look at the sugars on the Nutrition Facts panel. If the food provides more than 10 grams of sugar per serving, that's going to be about half of all the added sugar a woman can eat in a day. One note: Not all food packages break out added sugars from total sugar (some sugar occurs naturally in food, like

Not So Sweet: Top Sources of Added Sugar

Everyone knows how sugary sodas are, so it's no surprise that they're the leading source of added sugar in the U.S. diet. But you may be shocked to learn the other foods that made the list. If you're looking to drop a few dress sizes, you should definitely avoid making these an everyday menu item:

FOOD OR BEVERAGE	PERCENT CONTRIBUTION TO TOTAL ADDED SUGAR INTAKE
Regular soft drinks	33%
Sugars and candy	16%
Cakes, cookies, pies	13%
Fruit drinks	10%
Dairy foods (sweetened yogurt, ice cream)	8.5%
Cereals and breads (cinnamon toast, sweetened cereals)	6%

Source: Guthrie JF, Morton JF. Food Sources of added sweeteners in the diets of Americans. J Am Diet Assoc. 2000 Jan; 100 (1): 43–51.

fruit juice, milk, and plain yogurt). Look at the ingredient list to see whether the source of the sugar is added or naturally occurring.

How can you tell? If any of these are among the first three ingredients, the food is sugar-rich: brown sugar, corn sweetener, corn syrup, sugar (dextrose, fructose, glucose, sucrose), sorghum, high-fructose corn syrup, honey, invert sugar, malt sugar, molasses, raw sugar, syrup, agave, brown rice syrup, or maltodextrin.

You're just three quick steps from filling your cart with the healthiest picks.

FAT HABIT #48

With my schedule, I don't have time to cook. —MOLLY P.

This is often more of a prioritizing problem than a scheduling one. It's not that you don't have the time—it's that you haven't made your health a priority. When you really think about it (and be honest with yourself), you can probably find a way to free up twenty or thirty minutes in your day to shop and/or cook a healthy meal.

For the most part, the busiest people we know (including some CEOs) have the healthiest habits: They find time to eat right and get daily exercise. It's not that they have any more free time than anyone else (in many cases, they have more demands and less time). It's that they've made their health a priority.

Once you make the switch—thinking of healthy eating as a must on your to-do list—you'll find that the thought of ordering in or going to a restaurant will feel like a bigger hassle than whipping up a healthy meal yourself. In fact, you could have a nutritious meal on the table in less time than it takes to dial for delivery.

SLIM SOLUTIONS

If your to-do list is testing the memory capacity of your smartphone, we can help. The good news is that eating healthfully doesn't have to take a lot of time or effort. With a little forethought and planning, making your own meals and snacks is a snap. How much time do you need to eat a container of Greek yogurt with a piece of fruit for breakfast? Or a pita stuffed with hummus and veggies for lunch? Probably less time than you spent standing in line for your latte.

Use the following tips to simplify your meals and snacks.

MAKE THE MOST OF YOUR WEEKENDS

Planning healthy meals and snacks is the part that will take the most time, and we recommend that you do this over the weekend, preferably on Sunday night, when you have recovered from your busy week.

BUILD YOUR QUICKIE RECIPE REPERTOIRE

Aim to have two to three go-to recipes that take no more than fifteen minutes to make. And try to have the ingredients for them readily available, so if there's a day where you just can't think of what to make or are short on time, you can revert to one of these quick and easy solutions.

COOK IN BIG BATCHES

Double your recipes so that you can have plenty of leftovers in the refrigerator or freezer for future use. It may take a little more time in the beginning, but it will save you in the long run—in terms of both time and calories.

USE LEFTOVERS AS MAKE-AHEADS

Whenever we cook, we try to use leftover ingredients the next day in another dish. Search online for "cook once, eat twice" ideas, like making salmon steaks one night, then making salmon patties out of the leftovers another day. Better yet, ensure that you have leftovers by making extra. If you're whipping up grilled chicken for dinner, double the chicken so you have some to add to a salad or for another chicken dish the next day.

STOCK UP ON FROZEN MEALS

Head to the freezer section to find a calorie-controlled frozen dinner that can serve as the foundation for a meal. Look for those that have less than 350 calories and provide veggies, lean protein, and whole grains. Add some additional veggies, salad greens, or some fresh fruit, and you've got a healthy, balanced meal that's a cinch to make. Stash a few of these meals in your freezer for those no-time-to-cook nights.

CUT OUT PREP

Buy a veggie party tray at your local supermarket and use those precut and prewashed veggies during the week. You'll be more likely to eat them if they're ready to go. You can also use prewashed and bagged salads to save time, or if your supermarket sells them, you can opt for an individual salad. Top with your own dressing and you have a solid foundation for lunch or dinner.

CRACK ONE OPEN

Eggs, that is. Eggs are protein-rich and relatively low in calories, so we use them a lot for breakfast, lunch, and dinner recipes. One of Julie's fastest meals is her Spinach, Mushroom, and Onion Frittata. It takes less than fifteen minutes from start to finish and is an excellent dinner that provides leftovers for breakfast or lunch.

STICK WITH SALAD

Another great idea is to make a big salad for a one-dish dinner. Julie calls these "kitchen-sink salads" because she throws everything in them—minus the kitchen sink. Use whatever greens you want; then pile on cut veggies, hard-boiled eggs, lean protein like chopped grilled chicken breast or lean beef, and some toasted seeds. Serve your salad with whole-grain bread or rolls, or brown rice.

DO A DELI DINNER

Julie swears by her supermarket deli for piecing together last-minute meals. She often picks up a rotisserie chicken and a roasted veggie or beet-salad side dish. A serving of lean protein, one or two veggie side dishes, and a ninety-second package of wild or brown rice equals one quick meal. Even though you didn't cook it, you assembled it, and that's going to be better than stopping at your local fast-food outlet, ordering pizza, or going to a restaurant. (For more of our favorite quick, easy, and nutritious recipes, see Chapter 9.) And in most cases, you can find out the nutrition info of the foods; simply ask the store manager.

FAT HABIT #49

I don't know how to cook—at all. —JESSICA A.

Do you feel more comfortable doing your own taxes than cooking? You're not alone. One recent survey found that 28 percent—almost one-third—of American adults said they don't know how to cook. The average American now spends less than a half hour per day cooking. That's about the same amount of time as one episode of *Top Chef.* Speaking of cooking shows, we've become a nation of armchair chefs who'd rather watch Paula Deen, Jamie Oliver, Mario Batali, or Rachael Ray cook on TV than step into the kitchen ourselves.

Cooking is not a spectator sport. It's something that everyone can—and should—do, and it doesn't have to be complicated or time-consuming. There's really nothing to it, other than doing it. And the benefits are too many to list. To name just a few: It can boost self-confidence, save you cash, improve your health and overall diet, and, last but not least, help you lose weight.

SLIM SOLUTION

All you really need to get started: a few basic recipes. Where to find them? Check out our list of cookbooks and websites written by registered dietitians or other experts with a strong nutrition focus, below. These are all pretty basic—you won't be deboning chickens, deglazing pans, or making any béarnaise sauces or stuffed squabs.

Still have questions? No problem! You have a personal cooking school right at your fingertips. Google any recipe or cooking technique, and you'll get loads of results with step-by-step instructions. We often access videos for various cooking techniques. Things we've searched: "How to zest a lemon," "How to sharpen a chef's knife," and "How to strain yogurt."

BOOKS TO BUY

How to Cook Everything: The Basics, by Mark Bittman (Wiley, 2003).
Designed to give you confidence in the kitchen, this cookbook features easy-to-follow directions for making virtually everything. Not only will you whip up some of the best food you've ever eaten, you'll save money and eat more healthfully too.

Lickety-Split Meals for Health Conscious People on the Go!, by Zonya Foco, RD (ZHI Publishing, 2007).
This is a great resource with 175 deliciously healthy recipes and pages of nutrition, fitness, and grocery tips. Plus, it has a wipe-erase menu planner included.

The Complete Idiot's Guide to 200-300-400 Calorie Meals, by Heidi Reichenberger McIndoo, MS, RD, LDN, and Ed Jackson (Alpha Books, 2012).
If you're looking for healthy, delicious recipes and menus created with real, whole foods, this is the book for you. There's nothing

artificial—just wholesome ingredients put together to create hundreds of meals and snacks to keep you healthy, happy, and satisfied.

Quick & Healthy Recipes and Ideas, by Brenda Ponichtera, RD (Small Steps Press, 2008).
This cookbook includes more than two hundred recipes, sample menus, and grocery lists, as well as what to add to recipes to complete meals.

The 400 Calorie Fix Cookbook: 400 All-New Simply Satisfying Meals, by Liz Vaccariello with Mindy Hermann, RD (Rodale, 2011).
We recommend 400-calorie meals in our meal plans, and this book provides enough options that you'll never get bored. Each recipe includes suggested sides that you can add to create a balanced meal.

Cooking Light Fresh Food Fast: Weeknight Meals: Over 280 Incredible Supper Solutions (Cooking Light/Oxmoor House, 2010).
This cookbook is great because the recipes take just minutes to prepare and have no more than five ingredients. They also have options for two, four, or six servings, with full nutritional analyses of every recipe.

The EatingWell Healthy in a Hurry Cookbook: 150 Delicious Recipes for Simple, Everyday Suppers in 45 Minutes or Less, by Jim Romanoff and the editors of *EatingWell* (Countryman Press, 2006).
This book contains some of the best of *EatingWell* magazine's quick and easy recipes. The cookbook is filled with beautiful photographs of dishes and will quickly become your go-to when time is tight.

Clean Eating for Busy Families: Get Meals on the Table in Minutes with Simple and Satisfying Whole-Foods Recipes You and Your Kids Will Love, by Michelle Dudash, RD (Fair Winds Press, 2012).
If you want dietitian-approved, family-friendly meals, this cook-

book is a great option. The focus is on natural, wholesome ingredients, which are transformed into great meals. Most of the recipes in the book take less than thirty minutes to make.

1,000 Low-Calorie Recipes, by Jackie Newgent, RD (Wiley, 2012). This incredible cookbook is packed with tasty, diet-friendly dishes that the whole family will love. The recipes are all less than 500 calories (many less than 300 calories) and give you plenty of variety.

SITES TO BOOKMARK

CookingLight.com

At CookingLight.com, you'll find healthier twists on classic recipes, along with nutrition, fitness, and health features.

EatingWell.com

Like CookingLight.com, this site is a great resource for healthy recipes, as well as nutrition and health feature articles.

SkinnyTaste.com

This is one of our favorites, because Gina includes wonderful photos that take you step by step through each of her flavor-rich, calorie-poor recipes.

SkinnyKitchen.com

At SkinnyKitchen.com, you'll find many of your favorite comfort foods, like chicken pot pie, fried chicken, and mashed potatoes, skinnyfied. We also like the great food photography that's included with each recipe.

FAT HABIT #50

I'd eat a lot more fruits and veggies, but I can't afford organic.

—CHERYL G.

It's true: Organic foods (those that meet USDA organic criteria, which includes no synthetic chemicals, irradiation, sewage sludge, prohibited pesticides, genetically modified organisms, etc.) are more expensive than conventional. In fact, they can be anywhere from 20 to 100 percent more expensive; the priciest organic picks are meat, poultry, and dairy products. That's primarily because organic farm production costs are higher and crop yields are lower.

But you don't have to drop that kind of cash to eat healthfully. Research published in the *American Journal of Clinical Nutrition* that looked at some fifty years of organic research came to the conclusion that there is no significant nutritional difference between conventional and organic crops and livestock. If there are any increases or decreases in nutrients like potassium, vitamin C, or omega-3s, they are so small that they don't make one a better pick than the other in terms of nutrition.

(Of course, there are still plenty of good reasons to go organic if you can afford it. For one, it's a more Earth-friendly way to eat. Also, by opting for organic, you can help limit your exposure to pesticides and other potentially harmful chemicals used to grow food.)

The bottom line: If you're not eating your five or more daily servings of produce—even conventional produce that may contain trace amounts of pesticide residue—you're cheating your health.

SLIM SOLUTIONS

PICK AND CHOOSE

You don't have to opt for organic for *any* produce—you can get rid of most pesticide residue with a good washing. Still, there are some produce picks that are typically higher in pesticide residue than others. If you had some extra money that you were willing to put toward your grocery bill, this would be the perfect way to spend it.

Thanks to the Environmental Working Group (EWG), a non-profit consumer watchdog group dedicated to environmental agricultural issues, we know which picks contain the most pesticide residue. The EWG refers to these fruits and veggies as the Dirty Dozen. For these items, the price of organic or another alternative may be worth the added cost. One way to pinch pennies: Look for frozen organic options, which pack the same number of nutrients as (and sometimes more than) fresh, but are a lot less expensive.

THE DIRTY DOZEN

Apples	Imported nectarines
Bell Peppers	Lettuce
Blueberries	Peaches
Celery	Potatoes
Cucumbers	Spinach
Grapes	Strawberries

The EWG also lists the produce picks that contain the least amount of pesticide residue; these are called the Clean 15. You can save your cents and choose conventional for these fruits and veggies.

THE CLEAN 15

Asparagus	Eggplant	Onions
Avocados	Grapefruit	Pineapples
Cabbage	Kiwi	Sweet Peas
Cantaloupe	Mangoes	Sweet Potatoes
Corn	Mushrooms	Watermelon

Even when you're not buying organic, the cost of produce can quickly add up. Try these tips to increase your fruit and veggie intake without emptying your wallet:

BUY LOCAL AND IN SEASON

Be sure to hit your local farmers' market as soon as it opens. Seasonal foods not only taste better but often cost less as well. Think ahead and stock up on fruits and vegetables in their natural season in order to can or freeze them for the off-season.

JOIN A COMMUNITY-SUPPORTED AGRICULTURE PROGRAM

There are great community-supported agriculture (CSA) programs in many parts of the United States. When you join a CSA, you'll get weekly deliveries of in-season, locally grown produce. The prices are great and it will help you learn how to use a wide variety of produce. Local Harvest, a nonprofit association dedicated to sourcing fresh, local ingredients, allows you to find farmers' markets and CSAs in your area through their website, www.localharvest.org.

GROW YOUR OWN

You don't have to have a green thumb to plant some fruits and veggies in a backyard garden. Plants like lettuce, tomatoes, eggplant, and many others can be grown in small spaces. Have no yard? You can grow many of these in pots.

FAT HABIT #51

I never use a shopping list. —KAREN K.

Spontaneous shopping is a surefire way to sabotage your weight-loss efforts. Planning is half the battle—think of your shopping list as your weapon against weight, your protection against pounds, your buffer against blubber, your . . . Well, you get the drift.

When you create a shopping list, it reaffirms to yourself that you're committed to losing weight. Without it, you open yourself up to temptation ("Hmm, chocolate doughnuts? Sure, why not!") and excuses ("I don't have the ingredients to make dinner, so I might as well order in"). Create a list; stick to the list; own the list!

SLIM SOLUTIONS

MAKE YOUR LIST

Do it on the weekends, when you have more time to sit and think about your dinners for the next few days. Once you have a framework for what you're making, then you can start on your list.

CHEAT

Use the sample grocery list in Chapter 9, an online grocery list template, or any of the grocery list smartphone apps below. Remember, if you're new to cooking, your list may seem a bit overwhelming, because you need to get all the ingredients to stock your kitchen. Once you've been cooking for a few months, you'll notice that shopping becomes much more streamlined.

SHOPPING LIST: THERE'S AN APP FOR THAT

Shopping lists get a high-tech face-lift thanks to grocery list apps that you can download for your smartphone or tablet. While we're more old-school (yep, we still prefer the good old pen-and-paper approach), these apps can sync up to coupon sites and recipe websites so that your ingredients are automatically downloaded into your grocery list and much more. Here are a few worth checking out:

- **Grocery IQ.** This app is consistently rated as one of the best for creating grocery lists. You can choose from their database or use barcodes from products. It also allows you to share your list with others and find coupons for items on your list.
- **Grocery Gadget.** This app gets great reviews for what you can do with it, like linking multiple accounts to one list. One downside: It's not free, like many other grocery list managers.
- **ShoppingList.** This app features multiple shopping lists that sync across numerous devices, so if your husband is on shopping duty, he knows exactly what he should be buying.
- **ShopWell.** This app is set up to focus on healthy foods and purchases that meet your customized nutritional preferences (e.g., gluten-free, low-fat, low carb). You can also use the app while shopping to scan products to see whether they fit within your diet preferences and how they score nutritionally.

FAT HABIT #52

I can't afford to eat right—I usually go for inexpensive value meals.

—SARA P.

Fast-food or quick-serve "value meals" are far from a good deal. Sure, they might save you some cash in the short term, but they contribute to obesity and other costly problems in the long run. The fact is, you can't afford to *not* eat right.

SLIM SOLUTIONS

While you can certainly spend a lot to eat well, you don't have to. Our guide to good nutrition can fit even the most frugal budgets.

USE A SHOPPING LIST

You can save up to 40 percent at the checkout just by making a grocery list. People who make—and follow—a list avoid expensive impulse purchases and guess-buying things they think they need but really don't.

DON'T SHOP HUNGRY

This is obvious, but research shows that if you shop when you're starving, you'll buy more and be more likely to cave in to cravings. Eat a piece of fruit or some veggies with dip before heading to the supermarket to help cut down on unnecessary purchases.

LOOK FOR GENERIC VERSIONS

Many generic or store brands are made to similar specs of the category leader, so nutritionally they're usually equivalent but just don't have the same brand name and marketing hype.

COMPARISON SHOP

Use unit price tags (aka shelf tags), which are located on store shelves directly beneath products, to compare products. That way you'll know the price per unit, such as a fluid ounce for beverages or an ounce for cereals, and can see how it stacks up to other brands. For example, you can find store-brand cereals at $.13 per ounce, compared with Kellogg's individual-serving multipacks, which may cost around $.75 per ounce, or nearly six times more. If there's no nutritional advantage, you can save your money by choosing the store brand.

EAT MORE MEATLESS MEALS

Beef, poultry, and seafood are among the priciest items you'll buy. Eating vegetarian means that you'll eliminate some of these more expensive ingredients, and you can replace them with less expensive items like whole grains, beans, and produce. We recommend a meatless dinner at least once a week, but if you go meat-free several days a week, that's fine too.

SHOP AT THE FARMERS' MARKET

Farmers' market foods are often the best bargains, because they're in season. Plus, unlike supermarket foods, you aren't paying for the coast-to-coast transportation, packaging, and marketing of the foods.

FAT HABIT #53

I like to cook, but my recipes are so unhealthy. —REBECCA V.

It's great that you're cooking at home—and even better that you enjoy doing so. However, if your dishes contain blobs of butter, oodles of oil, and scads of sugar, you're not reaping the benefits of a home-cooked meal.

SLIM SOLUTIONS

LOG ON

It's time to think out of the box—the recipe box, that is. If your collection is full of diet-derailing dishes, get online. We often find excellent quick and healthy recipes at places like Cooking Light.com, MyRecipes.com, EatingWell.com, Health.com, Weight Watchers.com, and through many of our favorite commodity board sites, like the Hass Avocado Board (www.avocadocentral.com), the

California Strawberry Commission (www.californiastrawberries .com), the U.S. Potato Board (www.potatogoodness.com), and the USA Rice Federation (www.usarice.com), among others.

MAKE SOME MINOR MODIFICATIONS

You can significantly reduce the number of calories as well as the sugar and saturated fat in most recipes with three easy tweaks:

1. | *Perfect the portion.* Cut back on portion sizes. For example, if your cookie recipe says it makes two dozen cookies, make two and a half dozen from the same amount of cookie dough. If your lasagna is supposed to make eight servings, cut it into ten or more servings. Don't worry about skimpy servings—they're usually all too big to begin with, because recipes in cookbooks today serve up bigger serving sizes than ever before. One study found that many of the recipes in the same cookbook, *The Joy of Cooking*, increased serving sizes in each print edition over the past seventy years. Today's recipes are designed to satisfy the average overweight American, not someone trying to lose and maintain a healthy weight.

2. | *Cut back on fat.* You can generally cut about a fourth of the butter or oil in a recipe without affecting the outcome too much. With baked goods, try replacing some—not all—of the fat with fruit purees. Use low-fat or nonfat milk in place of full-fat; try non-fat or low-fat Greek yogurt instead of sour cream. When making recipes that call for meats (e.g., casseroles, pizza, pasta with meat sauces), use two to three times as many veggies as the dish calls for and one-fourth less meat. You can pump up the volume of your recipes with "free" veggies—they add fiber and satisfaction to your dishes without the extra calories.

Make Smart Swaps

Use our swapportunity chart below for more ways to lighten up your recipes.

COOKING AND BAKING SUBSTITUTIONS TO CUT CALORIES, SATURATED FAT, AND ADDED SUGARS	
RECIPE CALLS FOR	YOUR SWAPPORTUNITY
1 large egg	2 whites When baking, swap whites for only half of the eggs that the recipe calls for.
1 cup heavy cream	1 cup half-and-half
1 cup half-and-half	1 cup whole milk
1 cup whole or 2 percent milk	1 cup skim milk
½ cup sweetened and condensed whole milk	½ cup sweetened and condensed nonfat milk
1 cup evaporated milk	1 cup skim evaporated milk
1 cup sour cream	1 cup low-fat plain Greek yogurt or 1 cup fat-free or low-fat sour cream
1 ounce cream cheese	1 ounce light cream cheese or Neufchâtel cheese
1 cup shredded cheese	¾ cup shredded cheese
½ cup nuts	¼ cup toasted nuts
1 cup oil for baking	½ cup fruit puree and ½ cup oil
Butter or margarine to prevent sticking	Cooking spray with nonstick pans
1 stick butter	1 stick margarine/soft spread or ½ stick butter plus ½ soft spread
For quick breads, muffins: ½ cup sugar	¼ cup sugar plus 6 medium dates chopped
1 cup chocolate chips	½ cup mini chocolate chips
1 cup pasta	1 cup whole-wheat pasta or ½ cup pasta and ½ cup whole-wheat pasta
1 pound ground beef	1 pound extra-lean ground beef, ground skinless chicken, or turkey breast

Cooking and Baking with Olive Oil

Another swap we routinely recommend to boost the health of your diet—and ultimately your health—is using olive or canola oil in place of butter. This will work for most cooking methods, including roasting or sautéing. Use the chart below to figure out how much oil to use in place of butter.

When baking items like pies, cookies or light cakes, or anything with yeast, we recommend that you stick to what the recipe calls for, because oils don't work well in many baked goods. (One calorie-cutting baking trick: Julie makes quick breads, like banana bread and zucchini bread, and muffins with light olive oil or soft spreads in place of butter.) Eating home-made baked goods is just for special occasions, so you don't really need to find a substitute for butter.

BUTTER/MARGARINE	OLIVE OIL
1 teaspoon	¾ teaspoon
1 tablespoon	2¼ teaspoons
2 tablespoons	1½ tablespoons
¼ cup	3 tablespoons
⅓ cup	¼ cup
½ cup	¼ cup plus 2 tablespoons
⅔ cup	½ cup
¾ cup	½ cup plus 1 tablespoon
1 cup	¾ cup

3. | *Skimp on sugar.* If a recipe calls for a cup or more of sugar, you can generally get away with using only ¾ cup for every 1 cup. One caveat: You can't do this if the recipe is for candy or contains yeast.

FAT HABIT #54

I don't have any of the tools you need to cook. —EVAN R.

You don't need a kitchen that would make Martha Stewart jealous to whip up healthy, homemade meals. In fact, when you first start to cook, you need only a few basics. Trust us, we know—we both lived in New York City studio apartments, and barely had a countertop in our kitchens, let alone space for cookware, appliances, and gadgets. We got by with just the basics, and so can you.

SLIM SOLUTIONS

We asked expert chefs (who double as dietitians) what their most essential healthy kitchen items are. With fewer than fifteen items, you'll have all the tools you need to be a cooking connoisseur.

CRUCIAL COOKWARE

10- or 12-inch nonstick skillet: A large skillet is your workhorse pan in the kitchen. You can cook meats and poultry in it as well as eggs and veggies. Be sure the pan has handles that are oven- and broiler-safe.

Small 2- to 3-quart saucepan with lid: You'll get a lot of use out of this pan—you can cook rice, boil veggies, whip up soup, or make sauces with it.

Large 4-quart sauce pot: This is for boiling large amounts of pasta, soup, stews, or chili.

Jelly-roll pan: This is basically a cookie sheet with sides, which you can use to roast vegetables and chicken. You can bake with it too, of course.

NECESSARY KNIVES

No matter how much cooking you do, having the right knives makes it easier, speedier, and more enjoyable. There are only three knives that every kitchen needs:

Chef's knife: You can literally chop minutes off your prep with a good chef's knife. You want one with an 8- to 10-inch blade.

Paring knife: The paring knife is thought of as an extension of your fingers. You can use it for small jobs, like chopping and peeling fruit, or slicing up smaller produce, like shallots or mushrooms.

Bread knife: You need one serrated knife to handle bread and delicate (read: mushy) produce, like tomatoes.

WHEN BUYING A KNIFE, ASK YOURSELF THESE QUESTIONS:

Is the blade stainless steel?

Does it feel substantial, not flimsy?

Does the knife feel good in my hand?

GOTTA-HAVE GADGETS

Measuring cups and spoons: You probably can't eyeball two tablespoons of olive oil or a teaspoon of baking soda—and if some ingredients are off, you risk getting less-than-stellar results.

Stainless-steel grater: We like the stainless-steel box graters that have different hole sizes. The smaller holes are great for hard cheese, and the larger holes can be used to shred vegetables.

Whisk: Whisks help you beat eggs, make salad dressings, and much more.

Cutting board: Save your countertop and invest in at least a few cutting boards. Find a variety that are dishwasher-safe and have a nonskid surface for safety.

Blender: "A blender is ideal for pureeing soups and sauces, and with the addition of beans, you can make them creamy without adding any cream," says Jackie Newgent, RD, culinary nutritionist and author. "A blender also allows you to make velvety bean dips and hummus."

FAT HABIT #55

I always buy way too much meat, poultry, and fish,
so I end up with too much food. —MINDY H.

Feel like cooking—even when you're following a recipe—requires too much guesswork? It can be difficult to know how much meat (or any other ingredient, for that matter) you need to buy, because many recipes don't offer up easy ways of measuring ingredients.

So should you just guess? You may figure that it's easier to buy a little extra than have to make a special trip for an extra half pound of ground sirloin to finish off a meat loaf. But who wants to waste food . . . or the cash and extra calories?

SLIM SOLUTION

If you can do some quick math using our general guidelines, you can buy nearly exactly what you need. Figure that there's a 25 percent cooking loss in weight for most meats, fish, and poultry—so, 16 ounces of raw meat, fish, or poultry will provide about 12 ounces cooked, or four perfect portions.

For other common ingredients, use some of the handy cooking weights and measures below:

INGREDIENT WEIGHTS AND MEASURES

Apple	1 medium or 1 cup, sliced	6 ounces
Asparagus	16 to 20 stalks	1 pound
Bananas	1 cup sliced 1 cup mashed	1 medium or 2 small 2 medium
Beans, dried	5 to 6 cups cooked	1 pound dried (2¼ cups)
Bread	1 cup soft crumbs 1 cup dry crumbs	1½ slices 4 to 5 slices, oven-dried
Butter, margarine, or spread	2 cups ½ cup	1 pound 1 stick
Carrots	1 cup shredded 1 cup ¼-inch slices	1½ medium 2 medium
Celery	1 medium bunch 1 cup thinly sliced or chopped	2 pounds (11 inches) 2 medium stalks
Cheese—hard (such as blue, cheddar, feta, mozzarella, Swiss), shredded or crumbled	1 cup	4 ounces
Eggs, large whole	1 egg	¼ cup fat-free, cholesterol- free egg product
Flour	3½ cups	1 pound
Garlic	½ teaspoon finely chopped	1 medium clove
Lemons or limes	1½–3 teaspoons grated peel 2–3 tablespoons juice	1 medium 1 medium
Lettuce— iceberg or romaine	1 medium head 2 cups shredded 6 cups bite-size pieces	1½ pounds 5 ounces 1 pound
Meat, cooked (beef, pork, and poultry)	1 cup chopped or bite-size pieces	6 ounces
Mushrooms—fresh	6 cups sliced 2½ cups chopped	1 pound 8 ounces
Nuts (without shells)—chopped, sliced, or slivered	1 cup	4 ounces
Nuts (without shells)—whole or halves	3–4 cups	1 pound
Onions—green, with tops	1 medium 2 tablespoons chopped ¼ cup sliced	½ ounce 2 medium 3 or 4 medium

Onions—yellow or white	1 medium ½ cup chopped	3 ounces 1 medium
Pasta—macaroni	4 cups cooked	6–7 ounces uncooked (2 cups)
Pasta—noodles, egg	4 cups cooked	7 ounces uncooked (4 to 5 cups)
Pasta—spaghetti	4 cups cooked	7–8 ounces uncooked
Peppers, bell	½ cup chopped 1 cup chopped 1½ cups chopped	1 small 1 medium 1 large
Potatoes—new	10–12 small	1½ pounds
Potatoes—red, white, sweet, or yams	1 medium	5 6 ounces
Potatoes—red or white	1 cup ½-inch pieces	1 medium
Rice—brown	4 cups cooked	1 cup uncooked
Rice—parboiled (converted)	3–4 cups cooked	1 cup uncooked
Rice—precooked white (instant)	2 cups cooked	1 cup uncooked
Rice—regular long-grain	3 cups cooked	1 cup uncooked
Sugar—brown	2¼ cups packed	1 pound
Sugar—granulated	2¼ cups packed	1 pound
Sugar—powdered	4 cups	1 pound
Tomatoes	¾ cup chopped (1 medium) 1 cup chopped ½ cup chopped	5 ounces 1 large 1 small

I NEED AN EXTREME MAKEOVER—MY HOME IS MAKING ME FAT!

HOME: IT'S NOT JUST WHERE YOU HANG YOUR HAT. IN FACT, there's no place like home when it comes to packing on the pounds. Diet saboteurs lurk in every room of your humble abode, from your kitchen to your bedroom to your living room. Fortunately, you can turn your house into a health haven with a few simple slimming solutions. And changing your home environment can go a long way toward changing your waistline.

FAT HABIT #56

I get sucked into the TV. . . . I think I'm turning into a couch potato! —JENNY M.

Put down that remote and step away from the TV. The more time you spend watching television, the less time you have for just about everything else, including physical activity. It's a simple fact: Television monopolizes precious leisure time.

Think you can't spare even a few minutes to squeeze in a quick workout or make a healthy snack? Consider how much time we

Crazy-But-True Tube Facts

- Number of TV sets in the average U.S. household: 2.24
- Percentage of households that have at least one television: 99
- Percentage of homes with three or more TV sets: 66
- Percentage of Americans who regularly watch television while eating dinner: 66
- Number of hours of TV watched annually by Americans: 250 billion
- Percentage of Americans who say they watch too much TV: 49

Source: BLS American Time Use Survey, A. C. Nielsen Company, 2012

spend in front of the tube: According to the A. C. Nielsen Company, the average American watches four and a half hours of TV each day. That's about thirty-one hours per week, or two months of nonstop TV watching per year. Over sixty-five years, a person will have spent nine years glued to the tube. Just imagine what else you could have done during that time.

SLIM SOLUTION

Here's one piece of health and weight-loss advice that can benefit just about everybody: *Turn off your TV!*

When you veg out in front of the TV, you burn fewer calories than doing just about any other activity, including reading. In fact, it's nearly the calorie-burning equivalent of sleeping! Not to mention that you're more at risk for mindless eating as you unwind with an episode of your favorite reality show or sitcom.

If you unplugged, you'd have hours of extra time every day. You could use that time to cook a healthy meal, take a walk with a friend, go food shopping, or hit the gym. (If you decide to cut out

TV-Free and Loving It

After being virtually TV-free for about five years now, Katherine can say without a doubt that she doesn't miss it! But what about that great show that everyone's talking about, or that can't-miss sporting event? If there's something she really must see, she downloads it on iTunes or Netflix. She uses all that extra time to go hiking with friends, play with the dogs, or whip up a fresh meal from scratch.

all TV, you'll save at least $1,200 each year in cable bills too. A double bonus!)

Can't bear to say good-bye to your *Friends* reruns or take your last dance with the stars? Make a commitment to cutting your viewing time to less than five hours per week.

FAT HABIT #57

I like to fill up my plate—and my dishes are huge! —JANEL J.

Size *definitely* matters! Many standard entrée plates are 12 or even 14 inches in diameter. In your grandmother's day, plates were closer to 10 inches. You know what they say about big plates . . . big waists! On a 10-inch dinner plate, a portion of rigatoni looks like a meal, but on a 12- or 14-inch plate, it looks like you got cheated!

It's no coincidence that as plate sizes have increased, so have obesity rates. The more we put on our plate, the more we eat. One study found that 54 percent of Americans say they eat everything on their plate. The clean-plate club is one group you don't want to belong to.

SLIM SOLUTION

If your kitchen cabinets are filled with supersize serve-ware, it's time to downsize. This is one Slim Solution you'll really enjoy—who doesn't love a good shopping spree? And even better, this one's for your health!

Trading in for punier plates may seem like a cheap trick, but it's one that really works. Studies show that when your plate *looks* full, you're less likely to feel deprived, even though your portion size is smaller! Our decisions about eating often have little to do with how hungry we are. Instead, our brains tend to rely on visual cues, like the size of our bowls and plates, to tell us how much to eat. Large plates and bowls lead to more eating for one simple reason: They make portions look smaller.

Sure, new dinnerware may cost you some extra dough, but you'll more than make up for it in calorie savings. Studies show that going from a 12-inch plate to a 10-inch plate can reduce how much you eat by about 22 percent. The same is true for smaller bowls and spoons. Smaller serving spoons were found to result in a 14 percent decrease in food intake, while smaller bowls led to a whopping 50 percent decrease in eating.

While you're at it, why not splurge on some new glassware too? Choosing smaller, thinner glasses can help you slash calories. Research shows that you drink 75 percent more from a short, wide glass compared with a tall, thin one. (Better yet, skip calorie-containing beverages like soda, fruit juice, and iced tea altogether.)

FAT HABIT #58

*I like everything to match—including my
food and my plates.* —GENIE M.

It's not all about size—color counts too, when you're picking out plates. The color contrast between food and the plate it's served on can influence how much you eat. In one study, people who had a low food-to-plate contrast (for example, pasta with Alfredo sauce on a white plate, or pasta with tomato sauce on a red plate) served themselves 22 percent more than participants with high-contrast plates (for instance, pasta with tomato sauce on a white plate, or pasta with Alfredo sauce on a red plate).

The study also found that reducing the color contrast between the dinnerware and its background (e.g., table, tablecloth, or place mat) helps reduce overserving by as much as 10 percent. Use these findings to your advantage!

SLIM SOLUTION

To cut portions without "feeling" it, serve your food on dishes that have a high contrast in relation to the color of your food. Consider using a set of Fiestaware or other serve-ware that has multiple colors in a set, so you'll have many options. Want to eat less blueberry pie at your next book group meeting? Use a white plate. Employ the reverse strategy to help you eat more of the healthy stuff. Need to eat more greens? Serve them on a green plate!

FAT HABIT #59

*I can't stand to weigh myself. . . . I'm scared to even step
on the scale. I call it scale-itis.* —KELLEIGH T.

Have you been giving your scale the cold shoulder? Maybe you hid
it in some hardly used cabinet or banished it to the basement, where
it's now buried under a bunch of dust bunnies. You've convinced
yourself that knowing how much you weigh—actually seeing the
numbers on the scale in black-and-white—will totally deflate you.

If so, you have scale-itis, the word we use to describe total scale
avoidance.

Is avoiding the scale a bad thing? When it comes to weight loss,
the answer seems to be yes. Studies have shown that weighing yourself regularly—anywhere from once a week to daily—can help you
slim down.

SLIM SOLUTION

Make peace with your scale. Repeat after us: "The scale is my
friend."

Still skeptical? Consider the findings from the National Weight
Control Registry (NWCR). Those in the registry have shed at least
30 pounds and kept it off for more than a year, and some as long
as six years. NWCR members report weighing themselves frequently; 75 percent of participants weigh themselves at least once
per week.

Regular weighing can serve as an early warning system. When
you see you've gained a few pounds, you can then go into weight-
watching mode by paying closer attention to what you're eating or
evaluating your exercise routine. That way you prevent any further
gains.

The Right Way to Weigh

- **It's best to weigh yourself in the morning.** Food and beverages consumed throughout the day can weigh us down and lead to a higher reading in the evening.
- **If you're weighing frequently, remember that daily fluctuations in weight are common.** Just because you're heavier today than yesterday doesn't mean your weight control program isn't working. Look at the trend over weeks and months. Water retention during your period can add an extra pound or two.
- **The number on the scale isn't the only thing that matters.** How do you feel: stronger, healthier, leaner? Are your clothes getting looser or tighter? These nonscale measures can help keep you on track whenever there's an unexpected uptick on the scale.

One warning about weigh-ins: Frequent check-ins might not work for some people. If you know that you easily become weight-obsessed or you suffer from an eating disorder, it may be best to avoid the scale and use other ways to gauge your progress, such as how your clothes fit. (Talk to a health professional if you believe you have an unhealthy relationship with food and your scale.)

No matter how often you step on the scale, it's important to keep in mind that it's normal to have daily fluctuations in your weight. You shouldn't let the number on the scale affect your resolve or harm your self-esteem. Your scale can be a helpful tool on your weight-loss journey—along with other self-monitoring techniques, like keeping a food diary. As long as your weight is headed in the right direction over weeks and months, you're doing a great job.

FAT HABIT #60

Between work, family, and stress, I just can't get enough sleep.

—MAYA N.

Forget about counting sheep—you might as well start counting those extra pounds if you're having trouble nodding off at night. Over the last decade, researchers have found that skimping on sleep can lead to weight gain. One study published in 2005 followed the sleep patterns of eight thousand adults over several years. Those who slept fewer than six hours a night were more likely to be overweight or obese compared with those who got at least seven hours of sleep on most nights.

In 2009, a University of Chicago study concluded that participants consumed more calories from snacks and carbohydrates after five and a half hours of sleep than after eight and a half hours. Another study published in the *American Journal of Clinical Nutrition* found that after a night of abbreviated sleep, adults consumed more than 500 extra calories (roughly 22 percent more) than they did after eight hours of sleep.

Bouts of little or no sleep appear to disrupt the balance of appetite-regulating hormones—they boost the hunger hormone ghrelin and suppress our fullness hormone, leptin. That's like a double diet whammy: You're hungry, and you crave quick calories from foods like carbohydrates and fats.

Don't worry; you're not alone. You and another sixty million Americans are in the same sleepless boat.

SLIM SOLUTIONS

Aim for at least seven (if not eight) hours of shut-eye every night. Impossible, you say? Try these tips to make your bedroom a sleep haven:

STAY ON SCHEDULE

Try to go to bed and wake up at the same time every day, even on weekends, holidays, and days off. Having a regular sleep schedule reinforces your body's sleep-wake cycle and helps promote better sleep at night.

SKIP LATE-NIGHT NIBBLING

Avoid eating right before bed. This can cause indigestion, which can interfere with sleep (both falling asleep and staying asleep). If you must have a bite before bed, see Slim Solutions for Fat Habit #61. And, contrary to popular belief, a nightcap is not the best way to unwind before bed. While a drink may initially make you drowsy, too much alcohol can actually interfere with sleep. And way too much can lead to a hangover.

CREATE A SLEEP CAVE

The recipe for the perfect sleep environment consists of three ingredients: coolness, darkness, and quiet. If necessary, get blackout shades, a fan or "white noise" machine, even earplugs to set yourself up for sleep.

And don't skimp on a good mattress and pillow. Make sure you find ones that are comfortable for you.

NIX NAPPING

Long naps during the day can interfere with nighttime sleep—especially if you're struggling with insomnia or poor sleep quality at night. If you choose to nap during the day, limit yourself to about ten to thirty minutes, and try to do it midafternoon.

If you work nights, this rule doesn't apply to you. To make sure you get good sleep, keep your window coverings closed so that sunlight—which adjusts your internal clock—doesn't interrupt your daytime sleep.

INCREASE YOUR ACTIVITY

Regular physical activity can promote better sleep, helping you to fall asleep faster and to enjoy a deeper sleep. Timing is important, though. If you exercise too close to bedtime, you might be too energized to fall asleep. If this seems to be an issue for you, exercise earlier in the day.

FAT HABIT #61

When it's nighttime, I raid the kitchen. I'm a nighttime nosher.

—EILEEN B.

Nighttime nibbling is one of the worst Fat Habits (it's right up there with another p.m. pitfall: Fat Habit #60, "Between work, family, and stress, I just can't get enough sleep"). And unfortunately, it's all too common: More people are staying up late and eating in front of screens—whether they're shopping online, playing Words with Friends, monitoring their fantasy leagues, or hanging out with Jimmy Kimmel.

Studies show that people who eat the bulk of their calories in the evening are more likely to be overweight compared with adults who eat the majority of their calories when it's light out. In fact, the researchers found that eating past eight p.m. was an *independent* predictor of body weight and was correlated with total daily energy consumption, regardless of what time subjects went to bed or how many hours they slept.

Our body is programmed to eat during the day, when we're awake and most active, thanks to our hormones and circadian clock. Our late-night nibbling is driven by habit, not hunger.

Although some weight-loss experts argue that a calorie is a calorie—it doesn't matter when it's eaten—new research indicates that nighttime calories may be more detrimental. That's because they disrupt the hormones that regulate appetite and hunger, making it harder to lose and maintain a healthy weight. In fact, studies show that rodents get fatter when they're fed at times when they'd normally be at rest. Even feeding animals at different light-dark cycles results in weight gain. Night eaters may also be distracted when munching and crunching, and this too can lead to overeating. Another strike: The foods readily available and most appealing when it's dark out—chips, ice cream, cookies—aren't exactly the healthiest.

SLIM SOLUTIONS

Skip the nighttime feeding frenzy. You don't need to fuel up to fall asleep. You can put an end to late-night nibbling with these tips:

- *Fill up during the day.* If you're hungry at night, it may be that you're not eating enough throughout the day. "After dinner, you may try to make up for the lack of calories—and then some," say Lyssie Lakatos, RD, and Tammy Lakatos Shames, RD, the Nutrition Twins. Make sure you're eating a healthy, balanced breakfast and lunch, and a snack or two, if needed.
- *Eat a fiber-rich dinner.* Fiber keeps you full through those easy-to-cave-in evening hours, so you can withstand that intense urge to snack. Start your dinner with either a hearty nonstarchy vegetable soup or a large tossed vegetable salad, and drink plenty of water throughout the meal.
- *Delay your dinner.* Consider starting dinner an hour later, say seven instead of six. This leaves you less awake time to snack.
- *Don't let junk in the door!* Why test your willpower? Instead of torturing yourself by stocking your cabinets with lots of tempting treats, leave them at the supermarket. If it's unavailable, you

can't eat it. For tips on what to allow into your home, see Chapter 4 on grocery shopping.

- *Preplan your p.m. snack.* Planning is power. In fact, people often "crave" what they've planned for. Use that power for good by scheduling a healthy snack for yourself. Cynthia Sass advises, "Rather than spontaneously grabbing what's on hand, decide, by lunchtime, what you're having for dinner and as an evening snack and stick to it. Make it something satisfying enough to look forward to, but healthy enough to avoid calorie overload, like a parfait made from nonfat organic Greek yogurt seasoned with cinnamon, toasted rolled oats, and fresh in-season fruit, garnished with chopped nuts or dark chocolate chips. This 'think ahead' strategy is like deciding what to wear to work the night before—it just makes sense and works. In a nutshell, planning prevents chaos."

- *Stretch out your snack.* Choose foods that take a little time to eat. Katharine's favorite slow snacks: 2 cups of air-popped popcorn topped with 1 tablespoon of Parmesan cheese; nonfat Greek yogurt with ¼ cup of berries; or ½ cup of low-fat cottage cheese with ¼ cup of pineapple cubes.

- *Create an eating cutoff.* After you eat your nighttime snack, make it difficult to go back for more. How? Tell yourself the kitchen is closed and turn off the light. Then brush your teeth to signal that you're finished eating, the Nutrition Twins recommend. "That also helps distract your taste buds," say Lyssie Lakatos and Tammy Lakatos Shames.

- *Keep yourself busy.* Nothing kicks a craving into high gear like boredom. Fill your after-dusk downtime with other projects or tasks, like knitting, drawing, solving a puzzle, or exercising, instead of having a snack attack. Cynthia Sass urges, "Cut back on TV, which is a major trigger for mindless eating." Check your e-mail, do crunches or push-ups, jump rope, plan your calendar for the rest of the week, make that call to your mother-in-law that you've been putting off, etc. It's also a great idea to get out of the house a few nights each week. Take a nighttime yoga, dance, or Spin class; find a local book club or card game to join. Being active and being social is better than bingeing any day.

FAT HABIT #62

Breakfast? Who needs it? Coffee is my breakfast. —KATE M.

Are you a member of the "no-breakfast club"? If you run out the door with only a cup of joe because you're short on time or just can't stomach a morning meal, you could be in for real trouble. Here's why:

Eating breakfast is a key component to losing weight and maintaining weight loss. In fact, it's a daily habit for the vast majority of "successful losers" who belong to the National Weight Control Registry. A whopping 78 percent of them reported eating breakfast every day—and almost 90 percent reported eating breakfast at least five days a week.

Studies confirm the slimming benefits of breakfast. One recent Australian study found that children and adults who skipped breakfast had waist measurements that were nearly 2 inches greater than their breakfast-eating peers. The breakfast skippers also had higher insulin levels and elevated total and LDL (bad) cholesterol levels compared with those who ate a morning meal. Several other studies suggest that breakfast can affect our hormones and neurotransmitters.

But before you grab that day-old doughnut, keep in mind that some breakfasts are better than others. That dried-up baked good would crumble against a veggie-packed omelet. Protein seems to be key—a *protein-based* breakfast may help manage cravings and calories. A study published recently in the journal *Obesity* added to the growing scientific literature showing that eating more protein at breakfast can help you eat less at your next meal and reduce cravings for "unhealthy" foods.

SLIM SOLUTION

Start your day with a high-protein breakfast. It may help tame hunger, temper the brain's food-reward pleasure centers, and result in a healthier weight.

The solution here is a simple one: Eat breakfast every day. They don't call it the most important meal of the day for nothing. And try to start off with a healthy bite—it may help establish your hormonal appetite regulation system for the day. A scone or muffin with coffee won't quell your cravings as much as a protein-rich egg (6 grams of protein per one 70-calorie medium egg) or egg-whites breakfast (the protein is split between the yolk and white, but the white is lower in calories). Other stellar starters: oatmeal with peanut butter or yogurt (especially Greek yogurt); yogurt or cottage cheese with fruit; nut butters with a protein-rich whole-grain bread. If you're eating cold cereal, look for brands that provide at least 6 grams of protein per serving, and have it with a cup of skim or 1 percent milk to add an additional 10 grams of protein.

FAT HABIT #63

We serve our meals family-style. —JOANNE C.

Here's a quick pop quiz (don't worry—you don't have to study to ace this one). In which situation are you likely to eat more: when large plates of delicious food are placed on the table just inches in front of you, or when the food is left on the stove or counter and you have to get up to get seconds or thirds? Of course, the answer is when it's right in front of you.

This seems pretty obvious, but believe it or not, researchers have actually studied it. One group found that men ate 29 percent more food when a serving dish was on the table versus the counter; women ate about 10 percent more.

Family-style dinners play to our laziness and our desire to not call attention to ourselves (someone might notice you're having another helping when you get out of your chair as opposed to sneaking a scoop from the bowl beside you).

Think you're too smart to fall for the family-style food fest? Think again. Your brain is unbelievably unreliable when it comes to keeping track of intake. In one study, researchers videotaped people eating family-style and then asked them how many servings they thought they had consumed. Invariably, they reported eating only one or two. When the videotape was played back, it showed that they had eaten four servings!

SLIM SOLUTION

MOVE FOOD OUT OF ARM'S REACH

After all, out of sight, out of mouth!

This simple trick will give you an extra edge in the fight against extra servings. Research shows that simply seeing and smelling food can make you feel hungrier, even though you might feel full otherwise. Don't tempt yourself: Portion out your meal at the counter, and leave leftovers in the fridge.

Growing up, I was forced to clean my plate because "half the world was starving." —JANELLE S.

The logic in this age-old parental argument is severely lacking: How does cleaning your plate help world hunger? It won't. What it *will* do: make you fat.

As we already mentioned, many of us are eating off of oversize plates (see Fat Habit #57 "My dishes are huge!"). Plus, we suffer from "portion distortion," meaning we don't know what a moderate portion should look like anymore. This is partly because portion sizes in the United States have grown significantly since the 1960s, with the expansion of fast-food franchises. Portions grew there, and so did portions at home. Not surprisingly, our waistlines have followed suit.

SLIM SOLUTION

Don't have unfailing willpower? No problem. You can fool yourself full. Being aware of how environmental triggers (like the sight and smell of food or the size of your plate) can increase appetite is your first step. Then you can figure out how to work around them. As we discussed in Fat Habit #57, "My dishes are huge!", larger plates lead to larger portions. But using a smaller plate—around 9 to 10 inches in diameter—can help you feel more full on less food.

If you're not eating at home, remember that restaurants serve way more food than you need. Share with a friend, choose an appetizer portion, or ask the wait staff to pack up half the portion "to go" before your dish is served. See other tips for managing portions away from home in Chapter 6 ("I'm out of Control When out of the House").

I'm a "meat-and-potatoes" girl. And the meat
takes up half my plate. —JENNIFER L.

Are you still eating from the "old American plate"? You know—the
one that's filled with a huge slab of meat, a pile of mashed potatoes,
and maybe a sprinkling of peas? If so, it's time to enter the era of the
new American plate. Not only does portion size matter, but the proportion of different food groups matters too. The right proportion
of foods in a meal is not just important to overall health, it can also
make the difference between gaining or losing weight.

SLIM SOLUTION

RESHAPE YOUR PLATE!

If, for instance, you are having grilled chicken, broccoli, and mashed
potatoes, *half* of your plate should be broccoli, and only a *quarter*
each should be chicken and mashed potatoes. The basic formula:
Veggies or fruit should fill half your plate; on the other half, serve
yourself equal parts protein and starch.

I like to relax at night with a couple of glasses of wine. —JACKIE T.

An occasional cocktail is fine, but a multidrink nightly wind-down-
with-wine habit can easily interfere with your weight loss.

THERE ARE THREE BIG STRIKES AGAINST ALCOHOL:

1. | All alcohol is caloric and provides little, if any, nutritional
value. A couple of drinks each day can easily total more than 300
empty calories.

2. | Alcohol stimulates your appetite.

3. | Alcohol decreases your inhibitions, so the French fries, burgers, or pizza you might normally limit or avoid suddenly seem irresistible.

SLIM SOLUTION

LIMIT YOURSELF TO ONE DRINK PER DAY, OR TWO IF IT'S A SPECIAL CELEBRATION

Which adult beverage is the smartest sip? Use the quick reference guide below to help choose the most diet-friendly drink. Remember that mixers such as tonic water, fruit juices, and soda weigh down your glass with lots of added sugars and empty calories. If you're going with a mixed drink, ask for it to be mixed with diet soda or seltzer instead of tonic water. Avoid the supersize "specialty" cocktails that are commonly served at bars and restaurants in the summer—they can cost you more than 500 calories.

Ultra Light Beer (12 ounces)	55 to 65 calories
Light Beer (12 ounces)	100 calories
Rum and Diet Coke (1 shot distilled spirit)	100 calories
Wine (5 ounces)	120 calories
Wine Cooler (10 to 11 ounces)	120 calories
Vodka and Diet Cranberry Juice (12 ounces)	140 calories
Bloody Mary	140 calories
Gin/Vodka Tonic	200 calories
Rum and Coke	240 calories
Cosmo (5 ounces)	270 calories
Daily's Frozen Lemonade (10 ounces)	280 calories
Strawberry Daiquiri (6 ounces)	300 calories

FAT HABIT #67

I live in Miami and always have my AC running.
I like it cold in my house. —JILLIAN J.

Do you crank the air-conditioning? Beware: Chilling out may fill you out. Lowering your AC, on the other hand, could help you reduce feelings of hunger and cut calories (not to mention it can also help lower your electric bill).

It might sound crazy, but preliminary research suggests a link between the obesity epidemic and the increased use of air-conditioning over the past few decades. While the correlation between cooler temps and higher weight is not yet conclusive, there are some compelling theories on how air-conditioning could play a role.

Most homes and offices are now kept at a relatively constant temperature year-round, thanks to central air-conditioning and heating. This means your body expends less energy because it doesn't have to work to warm up or cool down, potentially leading to increased fat stores. People burn more calories when they're trying to maintain their body temperature at a comfortable level. Keep your house at 80 degrees and let your body do the work cooling you down to 70 degrees.

"I try to use as little AC as possible. Not only does it save money, but I feel better being a little warmer," Katherine says.

Another reason: Heat can put a damper on your appetite. Have you ever noticed on really hot days you're not as hungry as usual? That's because when you're hot, you're less inclined to dive into heavy, calorie-laden foods.

SLIM SOLUTION

Keep your house on the warmer side in the summer, about 76 to 80 degrees Fahrenheit, if you can stand it. This slight adjustment may increase the number of calories your body burns daily just to keep cool.

My kitchen's a mess—I don't know where anything is. —PAULINE T.

Lost your ladle? Misplaced your meat thermometer? You can't be healthy if you don't have control of your kitchen—a cluttered kitchen makes it that much harder to get excited about eating nutritious foods at home. So if you're serious about slimming down, you'll want to create an organized and inviting cooking and dining environment.

Why is eating at home so important for weight loss? Put simply, **home cooking equals healthier eating**.

Not only will making your own meals help you save calories and cut back on other harmful ingredients, it might also save your life. A recent study found that people who cooked up to five times a week were 47 percent more likely to still be alive after ten years. It's estimated that people consume 50 percent more calories, fat, and sodium when dining out. It's critical that you do everything you can to cook more at home, and it definitely helps to have a kitchen that's accessible and user-friendly.

SLIM SOLUTION

Having a fully stocked kitchen is only part of the equation of cooking success—you also have to know where everything is. Another key: storing nutritious foods in a way that encourages you to eat them—for instance, on a counter or low shelf as opposed to buried in the back of the fridge or stashed away on some high, hard-to-reach shelf.

Being organized will also help you keep track of which ingredients and equipment you have and which ones you need to buy. That way you'll always have on hand all of the basics you need to prepare healthy, delicious meals.

Ready to whip your kitchen into shape? Follow these tips:

1. | *Make room for healthy foods.* Is your fridge so jam-packed you can't even see into it? Are your cabinets so cluttered that stuff often flies out when you open them? It's time to do a quick cleaning and reorganizing. After all, the foods in your kitchen, where they're stored, and how accessible they are can all affect how much and how well you eat.

Start by tossing unhealthy items or putting them in places that are harder to see and reach. Also get rid of any expired foods. Reorganize the remaining foods, using the prime real estate in the fridge—accessible shelves and drawers—for healthy foods, such as vegetables and fruit and nonfat dairy. Do the same thing in your cabinets: Make sure you have a space front and center for the healthy stuff.

When putting foods away, store the items with the label and nutritional facts facing toward you. When you go to reach for the item, you'll be more inclined to check serving sizes and calorie counts to make sure you're doling out the right amount.

2. | *Store in style.* Another way to help organize your space is to invest in stylish, functional, clear storage containers. This will help you easily store cooked veggies, grains, poultry, fruit, and premade salads.

3. | *Organize utensils and cooking pots.* When you to cook or prepare healthy meals, you'll need to have your cookware and utensils handy. Colanders, spoons and spatulas, saucepans, a wok, pots and pans, a grater, a garlic press, and steamers should all be readily available.

4. | *Think ahead.* Prepare in advance healthy lunches, dinners, and snacks for busy weekdays. Think about what the coming week looks like, and aim to cook more balanced meals for yourself. You'll save cash (takeout and delivery aren't cheap), calories (remember, homemade equals healthier), and time (you don't have to rush to pack lunch in the morning if it's already made).

5. | *Create your own portion-controlled snacks.* Those 100-calorie snack packs can be a great way to enjoy a small amount of your favorite treats, but let's face it, they don't come cheap. Save some cash by creating your own: Buy your snacks in bulk and use your own containers to portion out your desired serving size. Store them in your pantry for easy access to a quick snack.

FAT HABIT #69

I put butter on just about everything. I know it's high in calories, but I just can't say good-bye to butter. —TAMMY C.

If "Pass-me-the-butter" is your middle name, listen closely. True, butter may add lots of flavor, but just 1 tablespoon has more than 100 calories and 7 grams of saturated fat (yes, that's the bad fat). So if you are baking with, cooking with, and slathering on the butter at every opportunity, it's time to reconsider.

SLIM SOLUTION

You don't have to eliminate butter entirely from your diet. Instead, switch to healthier and/or lower-calorie alternatives for *most* of your cooking and baking, and save real butter for the occasional treat. Don't worry; your meals will still taste amazing when you make these smart swaps:

- *Applesauce.* This ingredient is often used to replace oil in recipes, but it can also be a great alternative to butter, and works best in cakelike recipes. Replace half the amount of butter in your recipe with applesauce; if the recipe calls for 1 cup of butter, use ½ cup of butter and ½ cup of applesauce. If you don't mind a denser, moister bread, replace all the butter with applesauce to cut even more calories and fat.

- *Avocado.* Substitute half the amount of butter in a baking recipe with mashed avocado (it works well with cookies); use the same method as you would when using applesauce. It not only lowers the calorie content but also yields a softer, chewier baked good.

- *Trans fat–free spreads.* Use trans fat–free spreads in place of butter for your toast and muffins, or wherever else you might be tempted to use butter as a topping.

- *Canola oil.* In certain recipes, canola oil works as a great substitute for butter, especially if the recipe calls for melted butter. Although slightly higher in calories, it's much lower in saturated fat, cholesterol, and sodium.

- *Greek yogurt.* Replace half the amount of butter in your cookie recipes with half the amount of full-fat plain Greek yogurt. For example, if the recipe calls for 1 cup of butter, use ½ cup of butter and ¼ cup of yogurt. You'll reduce the calories and the saturated fat.

I'M OUT OF CONTROL
WHEN OUT OF THE HOUSE

If you think your home is loaded with diet hazards, wait until you step out the front door. Just when you think you've got a handle on healthy habits, you step outside and *boom!*—you're hit with a minefield of temptations that could easily lead you astray.

With thousands of fast-food restaurants, giant portion sizes, and clever marketing tactics that play on our emotions, we're more likely to eat more—even when we're not hungry!

Don't worry; you don't have to go into lockdown mode at home. This chapter will give you all the strategies you need to navigate the food world from the moment you set foot outside. We're not nutritionists sitting in an ivory tower, cooking meals from scratch every night, and eating a perfect diet. We're out in the real world facing the same obstacles and challenges as you. Katherine's lost more than a couple of battles involving chocolate and cupcakes staring her down from the local deli! And Julie is no stranger to corner-bistro carb cravings either. Here we offer you our top tricks and strategies for selecting the best dishes at restaurants, fast-food chains, your in-laws', airports, and everywhere in between.

FAT HABIT #70

I can't dine out without pigging out! —LIZ T.

In a perfect world, we'd all whip up every meal in our own kitchens, carefully controlling how much fat, sodium, and sugar we put into each dish. But that's just not realistic. Sometimes we must eat out due to business or travel demands. Not to mention that dining out can and should be one of life's greatest pleasures.

In fact, it's a pleasure that the vast majority of Americans enjoy: 82 percent of adults eat out at least once weekly. According to the National Restaurant Association, Americans spent about $1.7 billion at restaurants on a typical day in 2012.

Sure, we all know that restaurant dishes are loaded with calories, saturated fat, and sodium—but it's startling when you actually look at the numbers. Even appetizers and a seemingly healthy salad (when combined with dressing) can really cost you—about as much as an entrée when it comes to calories and fat. As many as one in four appetizers had calorie counts exceeding 1,100, according to a study by the RAND Corporation.

SLIM SOLUTIONS

The good news is that you can dine out without filling out by using the following strategies.

DON'T STARVE YOURSELF

When you know you're going out for dinner, do you try to save your appetite for that beloved entrée and dessert? Big mistake! The last thing you want is to wind up in a restaurant feeling starved. You'll be much more likely to choose high-fat foods and inhale them at record speeds. Instead, eat a normal breakfast and lunch. If you are dining out after six p.m., be sure to have a balanced snack before you go. (Check out the smart snack chart on page 79, "High-Protein Snacks Under 200 Calories," in Chapter 3.)

BYPASS THE BREADBASKET

If you're one of those amazing people who can have one slice of bread and stop (you're our hero!), you can skip this rule. For everyone else, you can save calories and fat by simply saying, "No, thank you," when the wait staff attempts to drop off a basket.

OPT FOR A HEALTHY APP

Get a healthy head start by choosing a good-for-you appetizer. A smart selection: salad. As we noted in Chapter 3, salads not only are a stellar nutritional pick but also help fill you up on fewer calories. Just be aware of caloric add-ons: Bypass bacon, skip the shredded cheese, say ciao to those croutons. Ask for dressing and/or sauce on the side, and instead of dumping it right on top of the whole dish, dip your fork in before eating each bit. This will impart the flavor of the dressing without adding too many calories.

Another slimming starter is a broth-based soup, like miso or chicken consommé. The high water content has been shown to result in a lower calorie intake for the whole meal. If a soup title features the word "cream" or "creamy," skip it!

PRACTICE PORTION CONTROL

Getting portions under control while eating out can be particularly tricky. First, plates and serving sizes are enormous. And second, we're assuming that you don't travel with measuring cups and spoons.

Fortunately, you don't have to try to force a food scale into your already packed purse. All you need in your eat-right arsenal are these handy tricks from Lisa Young, PhD, RD, author of *The Portion Teller Plan*, adjunct professor of nutrition at New York University, and nutritionist in private practice: "Order an appetizer or half-size portions instead of a full-entrée portion. Or you can share an entrée and a starter salad. This way you'll save calories and money! If these aren't options, never feel shy about bringing home leftovers. Ask your server to divide the serving in the kitchen, putting half in a doggie bag (ask to keep heated or cold if necessary) and plating the other half."

You may even find that half is too much for you. "I ask myself, 'How *little* do I *need* to get through the next three hours?'" says Tara Gidus, MS, RD, CSSD, LD/N.

"In other words, how much can I leave behind and still be satisfied for the next three hours?"

SPLURGE ONLY ON SPLURGE-WORTHY DESSERTS

"Unless there is some unbelievable, unique treat on the menu, do you really need another piece of chocolate cake or a brownie with ice cream?" asks Christen Cupples Cooper. Another approach: "Wait until you get home, and have a small bowl of ice cream or single portion of another reasonable treat. Chances are, you won't even want dessert when you finally get home." And even if you do, you'll likely consume far fewer calories.

FAT HABIT #71

I always order the "wrong" thing on the menu. —ALLIE S.

It's menu madness—there are literally dozens of dishes to choose from; some restaurant menus are more like novellas. And, of course, many of the options are total diet disasters. Don't panic. Simply put on your detective cap and sleuth out the slimmer options using these strategies (as well as the ones above in Fat Habit #70, "I can't dine out without pigging out!").

SLIM SOLUTIONS

BE PICKY ABOUT THE PLACE

When you choose a restaurant that offers plenty of healthy and delicious fare, you're already ahead of the game. In fact, this is probably 90 percent of the battle when it comes to eating out healthfully.

Fortunately, many restaurants have risen to the challenge: They're offering more nutritious dishes, and they've put their menus online to help guide your choice; some popular chains even make their nutritional information—including calorie, fat, and sodium content—available to consumers right at the restaurant. Take advantage of it: Do your homework so that before you even set foot in the door, you'll know what the healthy options are. Decide ahead of time what you're going to order, and stick with it.

SPEAK UP

Feel like a nudge when you have to make a special request or ask questions of your waiter? Keep in mind that you are the customer, and you have a right to order food the way *you* want it. Besides, restaurants have grown accustomed to catering to their health-conscious customers.

So don't be afraid to ask how something is prepared or cooked if you can't tell by looking at the menu, or request to have grilled chicken instead of fried on that salad. (Grilled is a tip-off that the dish is healthy, as is anything that's baked, roasted, boiled, or steamed.) These simple strategies could save you a significant number of calories and amount of fat.

Order Like an RD

Take a cue from clinical dietitian at Stamford Hospital Ilaria St. Florian, MS, RD: "Dining out is one of my all-time favorite things to do. I have a few dining guidelines that help keep me on track, though. For starters, if I am ordering a first course, I opt for a light garden salad instead of a heavy Caesar or wedge-blue-cheese-type salad. For the entrée, I choose fish or grilled chicken with vegetables and stay clear of steaks or pasta or anything that is served fried or with a cream sauce. For dessert, I satisfy my craving for something sweet by ordering a skim-milk cappuccino that tastes rich but is guilt-free."

Need more info on better-for-you menu choices? See our next Slim Solutions (refer to Fat Habit #72, "I love ethnic food").

Other special requests you shouldn't feel shy about making:

- Hold the butter.
- Put dressings and sauces on the side.
- Split the entrée portion.
- Instead of frying, make it grilled, baked, or poached.
- Prepare with minimal oil and salt.
- Skip the fries and replace with a salad or steamed veggies.
- Remove the skin from chicken.
- No chips, please!
- Tomato-based sauce instead of cream sauce.
- Broth-based soup only.

FAT HABIT #72

I love ethnic food. Chinese, Mexican, French—
you name it, I eat it! —ALEX K.

Here's a fortune that's sure to come true: If you love Chinese and other ethnic cuisine, you could easily be headed for diet disaster— no passport required! Just like typical American fare, the foreign foods you love could be either a diet boon or a diet bust. Where you eat and how you order can mean the difference between a genuinely healthy meal and an imported heart-attack-on-a-plate. Fortunately, we're here to help.

SLIM SOLUTIONS

Nutrition info is often not available for many ethnic eateries, so it's impossible to know exact stats for dishes. Still, it helps to go in knowing which dishes are typically better bets and which are calorie bombs. (Make sure to also use the tips from Fat Habits #70 and 71, above.)

MEXICAN

Better Bets

Caldo de Camarón—Caldo de Camarón is an authentic Mexican soup made with shrimp, potatoes, cilantro, and other spices.

Fajitas: chicken, shrimp, or veggie (with corn tortillas; skip the refried beans and request veggies).

Gazpacho—gazpacho is a tomato-based vegetable soup, traditionally served cold.

Pollo asado—a classic roasted chicken dish

Shrimp enchilada

Soft tacos: chicken, shrimp, fish, or vegetarian, if available. Most tacos come with cheese, cream, and guacamole. Ask for these on the side and use sparingly, and double up on veggies like lettuce, tomato, onions, and herbs like cilantro.

Tilapia plate

Limit or Avoid

Beef and cheese enchilada

Beef tacos

Carnitas

Chimichangas

Chorizo

Nachos with cheese

Quesadilla

Refried beans

Sopapillas

Tortilla chips

CHINESE

Better Bets

Chicken lo mein

Chicken with broccoli

Hunan tofu

Moo shu shrimp or chicken

Shrimp with broccoli

Shrimp with garlic sauce

Spicy green beans

Steamed brown rice

Steamed chicken and vegetables

Steamed vegetable dumplings

Steamed whole fish

Stir-fried seafood and vegetables

Stir-fried tofu and vegetables
Sweet-and-sour soup
Szechuan seafood
Vegetarian delight
Wonton soup

Limit or Avoid
Cold sesame noodles
Egg drop soup
Fried chicken and seafood dishes
Fried dumplings/wontons
Fried rice
Fried spring rolls
General Tso's chicken
Moo shu pork
Spare ribs

JAPANESE
Better Bets
Edamame
Hijiki (cooked seaweed)
Miso soup
Oshitashi (spinach with soy sauce)
Sashimi
Shabu-shabu (sliced beef, noodles, and vegetables)
Steamed fish
Steamed rice
Steamed vegetables
Sukiyaki chicken or beef
Sumashi wan (tofu and shrimp in a broth)

Sushi

Teriyaki: beef, chicken, or salmon

Yaki udon

Yakitori (chicken skewers)

Yosenabe (vegetables and seafood in broth)

Limit or Avoid

Fried bean curd

Fried dumplings

Tempura (Anything! Tempura dishes are always fried)

Tonkatsu (pork cutlet)

ITALIAN

Better Bets

Chicken cacciatore

Chicken marsala

Chicken or shrimp in wine sauce

Chicken piccata

Chicken scaloppini

Chickpea and pasta soup

Grilled calamari

Linguine with red or white (clam) sauce

Minestrone soup

Pasta primavera

Pizza with fresh veggie toppings

Roasted peppers

Shrimp marinara

Spaghetti with eggplant

Steamed clams

Limit or Avoid

Calzones

Cannelloni

Chicken, veal, or eggplant Parmigiana

Fettuccine alfredo

Fried calamari

Fried mozzarella

Garlic bread

Manicotti or ravioli filled with meat/cheese

Pasta carbonara

Pizza with pepperoni, sausage, or other meat toppings

Shrimp scampi

INDIAN

Better Bets

Aloo chaat (potato-based dish with traditional Indian spices)

Biryani: shrimp or veggie

Chicken and rice pilaf

Chicken or fish tikka

Chicken or fish vindaloo

Chutney

Coriander, tamarind, and yogurt-based sauces

Curried chickpeas

Dahl rasam

Gobhi matar tamatar (cauliflower with peas and tomatoes)

Lentils and spinach

Mulligatawny soup (lentil, veggies, and spices)

Matar pulao

Saag: chicken or fish

Shish kebab

Tandoori: chicken or shrimp

Tandoori roti

Limit or Avoid

Coconut soup

Curries made with cream or coconut milk

Fried samosas

Ghee (clarified butter)

Korma

Naan and kulcha (bread)

Pakora (fried dough)

Saag paneer (spinach with cream sauce)

FAT HABIT #73

I'm a sucker for McDonald's, Wendy's, Taco Bell, KFC. . . . If it has a drive-through, you can guarantee I'm driving through it! —GEORGE G.

Sometimes fast food is the only choice, and you know what? That's okay. Whether you think outside the bun, have it your way, or head for the border, you can probably find a pretty decent dish. Many fast-food joints have made significant strides in offering more healthful options—you just have to know how and what to order.

SLIM SOLUTIONS

THINK BEYOND BLACK-AND-WHITE

If it's a choice between fast food and skipping a meal, go ahead and eat something—but don't throw all caution to the wind. We know some people who reason that if they're at a fast-food restaurant, they may as well eat anything they want. Choose carefully.

SKIP SUPERSIZING

Opt for smaller sizes—even kids' sizes—of your favorite foods. That way you'll get a taste for far fewer calories and much less fat. This is especially true for fries, if you absolutely must have them.

SIP SMART

Choose a calorie-free or lower-calorie beverage, such as water or diet soda. Skip that shake!

DRESS THE PART

Select a low-fat or light salad dressing.

VEG OUT

Incorporate more veggies into the meal for extra nutrients and fiber. For instance, add a side salad or choose an entrée salad with lean protein.

DON'T BE FOOLED

Chicken isn't always better than beef. It can be—but not if it's fried or packed with cheese and bacon. In this instance, you'd be better off with a plain hamburger.

DON'T FORGET THAT CONDIMENTS COUNT

Hold the mayo—use mustard or ketchup instead to save calories.

STUDY UP

Ask whether the nutritional/calorie data is available so you can choose items with fewer calories and less fat and sodium. Many chains offer this information online, and some also have it in stores. Or keep a copy of the following chart with you (in your purse or car) just in case—that way you'll always be able to pick out the healthier options at popular chains.

HOW TO DO BETTER AT POPULAR CHAINS*

*Meals approximately 430 calories or less can be swapped for a main meal in Chapter 7 Meal Plan

	INSTEAD OF	OPT FOR	EVEN BETTER
ARBY'S	Max roast beef sandwich (580 calories, 22 grams fat, 45 grams protein) **Medium curly fries** (540 calories, 29 grams fat, 6 grams protein) **Regular Jamocha shake** (560 calories, 15 grams fat, 14 grams protein) *1,680 calories, 66 grams fat, 65 grams protein*	Super roast beef sandwich (430 calories, 17 grams fat, 23 grams protein) **Chopped side salad (dressing on side)** (80 calories, 5 grams fat, 5 grams protein) **Brewed ice tea (unsweetened)** *(510 calories, 22 grams fat, 28 grams protein)*	Roast chopped Farmhouse salad (dressing on side) (240 calories, 7 grams fat, 22 grams protein) **Water or brewed ice tea (unsweetened)** *(240 calories, 7 grams fat, 22 grams protein)*
BURGER KING	Whopper w/mayo (670 calories, 39 grams fat, 28 grams protein) **Large fries** (500 calories, 28 grams fat, 5 grams protein) **16-ounce soft drink** (150 calories, 0 grams fat, 0 grams protein) *1,320 calories, 67 grams fat, 33 grams protein*	Whopper Jr. w/o mayo (290 calories, 4.5 grams fat, 15 grams protein) **Small onion rings** (140 calories, 1.5 grams fat, 2 grams protein) **12-ounce (kid's) soft drink** (110 calories, 0 grams fat, 0 grams protein) *540 calories, 6 grams fat, 17 grams protein*	Tendergrill chicken sandwich w/o mayo (400 calories, 1.5 grams fat, 36 grams protein) **Side garden salad** (15 calories, 0 grams fat, 1 gram protein) **½ package Ken's fat-free ranch dressing** (30 calories, 0 grams fat, 0 grams protein) **Water or diet soft drink** *445 calories, 1.5 grams fat, 37 grams protein*
CARL'S JR.	Double western bacon cheeseburger (970 calories, 52 grams fat, 52 grams protein) **Medium fries** (460 calories, 22 grams fat, 7 grams protein) **Oreo cookie shake** (720 calories, 38 grams fat, 16 grams protein) *2,150 calories, 111 grams fat, 75 grams protein*	Kid's hamburger (460 calories, 17 grams fat, 24 grams protein) **Kid's fries** (250 calories, 12 grams fat, 4 grams protein) **Water or diet soft drink** *710 calories, 29 grams fat, 28 grams protein*	Charbroiled BBQ chicken sandwich (360 calories, 4.5 grams fat, 34 grams protein) **Side salad** (50 calories, 2.5 grams fat, 3 grams protein) **Low-fat balsamic dressing** (35 calories, 1.5 grams fat, 0 grams protein) **Water or diet soft drink** *445 calories, 8.5 grams fat, 37 grams protein*

	INSTEAD OF	OPT FOR	EVEN BETTER
DAIRY QUEEN	Crispy chicken sandwich (530 calories, 29 grams fat, 22 grams protein) DQ regular onion rings (470 calories, 30 grams fat, 6 grams protein) 16-ounce soft drink (150 calories, 9 grams fat, 0 grams protein) Peanut Buster Parfait (710 calories, 30 grams fat, 10 grams protein) *1,860 calories, 98 grams fat, 38 grams protein*	Grilled chicken sandwich (400 calories, 16 grams fat, 23 grams protein) Water or diet soft drink Small chocolate soft serve (150 calories, 5 grams fat, 4 grams protein) *550 calories, 23 grams fat, 28 grams protein*	DQ original burger (350 calories, 14 grams fat, 17 grams protein) Side salad, no dressing (45 calories, 0 grams fat, 2 grams protein) Water or diet soft drink DQ Fudge Bar (50 calories, 0 grams fat, 4 grams protein) *445 calories, 14 grams fat, 23 grams protein*
EL POLLO LOCO	Ultimate grilled burrito (650 calories, 20 grams fat, 38 grams protein) Tortilla chips (210 calories, 10 grams fat, 3 grams protein) 16-ounce soft drink (150 calories, 0 grams fat, 0 grams protein) *1,010 calories, 30 grams fat, 41 grams protein*	Original Pollo Bowl (540 calories, 4 grams fat, 38 grams protein) Pinto beans (140 calories, 0 grams fat, 9 grams protein) Water or diet soft drink *680 calories, 4 grams fat, 47 grams protein*	Flame-grilled skinless chicken breast (180 calories, 4 grams fat, 35 grams protein) Pinto beans (140 calories, 0 grams fat, 9 grams protein) Fresh veggies, no margarine (35 calories, 0 grams fat, 2 grams protein) Water or diet soft drink *355 calories, 4 grams fat, 46 grams protein*
KFC	Three-piece Crispy Strips meal (chicken plus cole slaw, biscuit, mashed potatoes, and gravy) (890 calories, 45 grams fat, 36 grams protein) 14-ounce (medium) soft drink (130 calories, 0 grams fat, 0 grams protein) *1,020 calories, 45 grams fat, 36 grams protein*	Oven-roasted Twister sandwich w/o sauce (includes lettuce/tomato) (330 calories, 7 grams fat, 28 grams protein) Cole slaw (180 calories, 10 grams fat, 1 gram protein) Water or diet soft drink *510 calories, 17 grams fat, 29 grams protein*	Roasted Caesar salad w/o dressing and w/o croutons (220 calories, 8 grams fat, 30 grams protein) Fat-free ranch dressing (35 calories, 0 grams fat, 1 gram protein) 2 percent milk or water (120 calories, 4.5 grams fat, 8 grams protein) *375 calories, 12.5 grams fat, 39 grams protein*

	INSTEAD OF	OPT FOR	EVEN BETTER
LONG JOHN SILVER'S	2 pieces battered fish (520 calories, 32 grams fat, 24 grams protein) 3 hush puppies (180 calories, 7.5 grams fat, 3 grams protein) Cole slaw (200 calories, 15 grams fat, 1 gram protein) 14-ounce soft drink (130 calories, 0 grams fat, 0 grams protein) *1,030 calories, 54.5 grams fat, 28 grams protein*	Fish sandwich (470 calories, 23 grams fat, 18 grams protein) Cole slaw (200 calories, 15 grams fat, 1 gram protein) Water or diet soft drink *670 calories, 38 grams fat, 19 grams protein*	2 pieces baked cod (240 calories, 9 grams fat, 44 grams protein) 2 Corn Cobbettes (180 calories, 6 grams fat, 6 grams protein) Water or diet soft drink *420 calories, 15 grams fat, 50 grams protein*
MCDONALD'S	Big Mac (540 calories, 29 grams fat, 25 grams protein) Medium fries (380 calories, 20 grams fat, 4 grams protein) Medium chocolate shake (580 calories, 14 grams fat, 13 grams protein) *1,500 calories, 63 grams fat, 42 grams protein*	Hamburger Happy Meal (burger plus small fries) (500 calories, 21.5 grams fat, 14 grams protein) Fruit-and-yogurt parfait (160 calories, 2 grams fat, 4 grams protein) Water or diet soft drink *660 calories, 23.5 grams fat, 18 grams protein*	Hamburger (250 calories, 9 grams fat, 12 grams protein) Snack-size fruit-and-walnut salad (210 calories, 8 grams fat, 4 grams protein) 8-ounce jug 1 percent milk (100 calories, 2.5 grams fat, 8 grams protein) *560 calories, 19.5 grams fat, 24 grams protein*
PIZZA HUT	2 cheese breadsticks (400 calories, 20 grams fat, 14 grams protein) Supreme Personal Pan pizza (710 calories, 34 grams fat, 32 grams protein) Water or diet soft drink *1,110 calories, 54 grams fat, 46 grams protein*	Veggie Lover's Personal Pan Pizza (560 calories, 22 grams fat, 24 grams protein) Water or diet soft drink *560 calories, 22 grams fat, 24 grams protein*	2 slices (from 12-inch) Fit 'n Delicious pepper, onion, and tomato pizza (300 calories, 8 grams fat, 12 grams protein) One trip to the salad bar for salad veggies only (60 calories, 0 grams fat, 4 grams protein—estimated values) Low-cal Italian dressing (35 calories, 0 grams fat, 1 gram protein) Water or diet soft drink *395 calories, 8 grams fat, 17 grams protein*

	INSTEAD OF	OPT FOR	EVEN BETTER
QUIZNOS	Regular Traditional Sub (450 calories, 8 grams fat, 29 grams protein) 1-ounce bag chips (150 calories, 10 grams fat, 2 grams protein) 16-ounce soft drink (150 calories, 0 grams fat, 0 grams protein) *600 calories, 8 grams fat, 29 grams protein*	Chicken Caesar Flatbread Salad (no bread, fat-free dressing) (440 calories, 4 grams fat, 32 grams protein) 1-ounce bag baked chips (110 calories, 1.5 grams fat, 2 grams protein) Water or diet soft drink *550 calories, 5.5 grams fat, 34 grams protein*	Balsamic Chicken Flatbread Sammie (170 calories, 3.5 grams fat, 11 grams protein) Side chopped salad w/fat-free dressing (125 calories, 0 grams fat, 0 grams protein) 1-ounce bag baked chips (110 calories, 1.5 grams fat, 2 grams protein) Water or diet soft drink *405 calories, 5 grams fat, 13 grams protein*
SONIC	Sonic cheeseburger w/ketchup (630 calories, 31 grams fat, 29 grams protein) Regular onion rings (500 calories, 28 grams fat, 6 grams protein) 20-ounce (medium) cherry limeade (230 calories, 0 grams fat, 0 grams protein) *1,360 calories, 59 grams fat, 35 grams protein*	Jr. cheeseburger (380 calories, 20 grams fat, 18 grams protein) Regular tater tots (220 calories, 14 grams fat, 2 grams protein) 20-ounce (medium) low-cal diet cherry limeade (15 calories, 0 grams fat, 0 grams protein) *615 calories, 34 grams fat, 20 grams protein*	Grilled chicken salad (310 calories, 13 grams fat, 29 grams protein) 12-ounce strawberry real fruit slush (180 calories, 0 grams fat, 0 grams protein) *490 calories, 13 grams fat, 29 grams protein*
SUBWAY	6-inch meatball marinara sub (560 calories, 24 grams fat, 24 grams protein) 1-ounce bag chips (150 calories, 10 grams fat, 2 grams protein) 16-ounce soft drink (150 calories, 0 grams fat, 0 grams protein) 1 chocolate-chip cookie (210 calories, 10 grams fat, 2 grams protein) *1,070 calories, 44 grams fat, 28 grams protein*	6-inch turkey breast sub (280 calories, 4.5 grams fat, 18 grams protein) 1-ounce bag baked chips (110 calories, 1.5 grams fat, 2 grams protein) 1 oatmeal raisin cookie (200 calories, 8 grams fat, 3 grams protein) Water or diet soft drink *590 calories, 14 grams fat, 23 grams protein*	6-inch Veggie Delite sub w/pepper-jack cheese (280 calories, 7 grams fat, 13 grams protein) 10-ounce bowl Spanish chicken/rice soup (110 calories, 2 grams fat, 6 grams protein) 1 package apple slices (35 calories, 0 grams fat, 0 grams protein) Water or diet soft drink *425 calories, 9 grams fat, 19 grams protein*

	INSTEAD OF	OPT FOR	EVEN BETTER
TACO BELL	Grilled Stuft chicken burrito (640 calories, 23 grams fat, 34 grams protein) Crunchy taco (170 calories, 10 grams fat, 8 grams protein) 16-ounce soft drink (150 calories, 0 grams fat, 0 grams protein) *960 calories, 33 grams fat, 42 grams protein*	Fiesta taco salad w/o the fried shell (470 calories, 24 grams fat, 23 grams protein) Pintos n Cheese (160 calories, 6 grams fat, 9 grams protein) Water or diet soft drink *630 calories, 30 grams fat, 32 grams protein*	Fresco ranchero chicken soft taco (170 calories, 4 grams fat, 12 grams protein) Fresco bean burrito (330 calories, 7 grams fat, 12 grams protein) Water or diet soft drink *500 calories, 11 grams fat, 24 grams protein*
WENDY'S	Single w/everything (430 calories, 20 grams fat, 25 grams protein) Medium fries (430 calories, 20 grams fat, 6 grams protein) 14-ounce (small) soft drink (130 calories, 0 grams fat, 0 grams protein) Small chocolate Frosty (320 calories, 8 grams fat, 9 grams protein) *1,310 calories, 48 grams fat, 40 grams protein*	Large chili (330 calories, 9 grams fat, 25 grams protein) Baked potato (270 calories, 0 grams fat, 7 grams protein) Buttery spread (50 calories, 5 grams fat, 0 grams protein) Water or diet soft drink *650 calories, 14 grams fat, 32 grams protein*	Mandarin chicken salad (including almonds but no fried noodles) (300 calories, 13.5 grams fat, 26 grams protein) ½ baked potato w/salt and pepper, no butter (135 calories, 0 grams fat, 3.5 grams protein) Water or diet soft drink *435 calories, 13.5 grams fat, 29.5 grams protein*

Note: Calorie, fat, and protein data current at time of publication

FAT HABIT #74

I'm obsessed with my bottom line (and I don't mean my derriere) when I eat out. I want to get my money's worth. —EMILY H.

News flash: Value meals may save you some dough, but in the long run, they'll end up costing you your health. These types of meal deals feature extra-large entrées, monster-size fries, and colossal cola.

Just take a look at the following chart to see the dramatic increase in portion size over the past sixty years or so:

SERVING SIZES THEN AND NOW		
FOOD OR BEVERAGE	1950S	TODAY'S PORTIONS
French fries	2.4 ounces	up to 7.1 ounces
Soda	7.0 ounces	12 to 64 ounces
Hamburger patty	1.6 ounces	up to 8.0 ounces
Hamburger sandwich	3.9 ounces	4.4 to 12.6 ounces
Muffin	3.0 ounces	6.5 ounces
Pasta serving	1.5 cups	3.0 cups
Chocolate bar	1 ounce	2.6 to 8 ounces

Order Like a Nutrition Pro

So what are we eating on the go? Here's a glimpse at some of our favorite menu options:

Julie: A chicken burrito bowl from Chipotle with brown rice, chicken, romaine, guacamole, and salsa. Also, a turkey sandwich without cheese with lots of veggies on whole wheat at Subway.

Katherine: Veggie on wheat with lettuce, tomato, spinach, green peppers, cucumbers, black olives, and American cheese from Subway. From Starbucks, I grab a Goat Cheese and Garden Veggies Bistro Box for a snack.

Christen Cupples Cooper: I opt for the following sandwich at a deli counter: two slices of whole wheat bread; turkey breast (some people ask for "less meat"; I ask for a regular sandwich and then take some meat off of it and save it for later—it's usually enough to make another sandwich); all the fresh veggies they have: lettuce, tomatoes, onions, olives, peppers, etc.; mustard.

SLIM SOLUTION

Saving pennies at the expense of saving your health is no deal. Repeat after us: Do not supersize! In fact, go the other way: Opt for the smallest portions available. At other restaurants, stick with the portion-control tips in Fat Habit #38, "I have no idea what a 'portion' looks like": Choose appetizer or half-size portions instead of a full entrée portion; share an entrée and a starter salad; and never be embarrassed to ask for a doggie bag so you can save half your meal for later.

Remember: A single restaurant meal may contain an entire day's worth of calories!

A small, 2½-ounce serving of French fries has 210 calories, compared with a whopping 610 calories in the 7-ounce size. While a 12-ounce soft drink contributes a relatively modest 151 calories to a meal, a megasize 42-ounce cup contributes about 529 calories. That's certainly a lot to swallow!

FAT HABIT #75

Food is my life—literally. I work every day with or around it.

—TIFFANY C.

How often do you think about food during the day? Around mealtimes, when you're reading your favorite cooking magazine or watching the Food Network, maybe when you're feeling stressed or bored? These thoughts can be dangerous—mental images of ice cream and thoughts of Twinkies make it hard to stay on track.

Now imagine if you had a job that involved food—maybe you're a chef or you work in a restaurant; perhaps you're a food writer or critic; or you might be a nutritionist or food purveyor. In these cases, food is on your mind all day long, and you may experience "phantom hunger phenomenon," feeling hungry when you actually aren't simply because you're around food.

SLIM SOLUTIONS

Kelly Weinhold, RD, one of our Appetite for Health contributors, offers tips for dealing with this job hazard:

GET UP

Whenever you can, get up and move; it's a distraction technique that will help get your mind off of food. "I'll go climb a few flights of stairs to grab a drink from the water fountain on another floor, or I'll find an excuse to go to the other end of the building," she says. Not only does it take her mind off hunger, but it also boosts her productivity.

DRINK H$_2$O

Ever confuse thirst and hunger? When we're not in tune with our bodies, it can be pretty easy to mistake the need for water with the desire for food. "If I think that my body might be dehydrated, I'll fill up my sixteen-ounce water bottle and take a few minutes to drink before actually turning to the food. Filling my stomach with fluid usually takes away that feeling of hunger, and I am able to continue with what I was doing."

MULTITASK

"Shifting my focus can usually help me forget that I thought I was hungry." Try making a few phone calls, responding to e-mails, or even organizing your desk or workplace. Getting the mind to reboot and refocus on something else will help you forget those phantom cravings.

CHOOSE A HEALTHY BITE

If you still feel that nagging hunger after trying the above tricks, then perhaps you really are hungry. Take a break from your work and devote fifteen to twenty minutes to eating something healthy. Focus on your food, not on all the other things on your to-do list, because multitasking while eating only leads to overeating.

Keep healthy snacks on hand that you can turn to for some quick energy. "Some of my favorites are plain yogurt with berries and granola, raw vegetables with hummus, a light-cheese stick and a can of low-sodium V8, and apple slices with natural peanut butter," she says.

FAT HABIT #76

I pig out on weekends! —JUSTIN G.

It's great to kick back after a long week at work, but be careful: That laid-back weekend mentality could spell trouble for your diet. In fact, if you're struggling to lose weight or maintain your loss, take a look at your weekend eating habits. A girls' night out, that romantic dinner for two, or a family barbecue often equals hundreds of additional calories above and beyond your weekday diet.

Most people who struggle with their weight gain at a rate of .17 pounds per week due to overeating on the weekends, according to researchers at Washington University School of Medicine in St. Louis. That's nearly 9 pounds gained in a year!

Saturdays prove to be the more difficult diet day—most individuals average about 200 calories more on Saturday alone—while Sundays seem to be our laziest day. That two-day combination of eating more and exercising less is a recipe for weight gain. Not surprisingly, subjects weighed the most on Mondays and the least on Thursdays.

SLIM SOLUTIONS

After a busy week, you deserve to blow off some steam and relax—but you still have to have some sense of control over your diet and exercise routine. Where to start? First, you have to be aware of common weekend diet wreckers; we've listed a few below. And then you need to devise a plan for dealing with each—once again, we're here to help. Check out our savvy solutions below.

SIP SMART

The extra glass of wine at dinner or a cocktail at a party can pack a major calorie punch. A 12-ounce beer contains 150 calories, light beer has about 100, a shot of a distilled spirit has 110 calories, and 5 ounces of wine has around 120 calories. Allow yourself no more than two drinks on each weekend night, and keep in mind that alcohol can stimulate your appetite and decrease your inhibitions ("Sure, I'll have a slice of that zillion-calorie cake") at the same time. When you drink, opt for lower-calorie cocktails, including ultralight or light beers and distilled spirits with seltzer or diet soda.

See more tips on alcohol in Fat Habit #78, "Beer, wine, sangria . . . bring it on!"

STAY ON SCHEDULE

No alarm clock, no meetings with the boss, no trains to catch—with no schedule to follow or no structure to keep you in line, it's easy to overeat. Many people need some sort of schedule to follow in order to stick to their normal diet. When they don't have one, they snack all day long.

So stick to your regular meal and snack times on weekends, and stay out of your kitchen when you're home to decrease the temptation. Another tip: Keep a journal to be mindful of what you're eating and why. . . . Are you even hungry? Probably not.

FIND NONFOOD REWARDS

You deserve a pat on the back for pulling off that presentation, putting up with your horrific boss, or volunteering at your local community center. But going crazy with your diet is not the best way to reward yourself. Indulging feels good only in the short term; long-term, it contributes to weight gain and can make you feel worse.

Instead, think about weekend "treats" that are non–food related. How about treating yourself to a massage or spa treatment, or a new group exercise class? They'll help you relax at a zero-calorie cost.

FAT HABIT #77

Call me Slurpie! When I'm out I can't get enough creamy coffee drinks, sodas, and smoothies. —RICHARD W.

You probably think before taking that extra helping of spaghetti and meatballs or an extra scoop of ice cream, but when was the last time you really thought, "Do I need to drink this?"

Researchers now know that by your beverage patterns alone, they can tell you whether you're at risk for becoming overweight or obese in the future.

Too many liquid calories are linked to overweight and obesity, type 2 diabetes, lipid disorders, and much more. In fact, liquid calories may inherently be much more damaging to our bodies than the same extra calories coming from solids, because liquids deliver their sugar and nutrients to the bloodstream more quickly than solids.

If your beverage is 100 percent sugar, it will cause blood sugar levels to spike as well as insulin levels. Do this too much and you'll quickly damage your health.

A recent beverage study found that nearly two-thirds of adults drink beverages with added sugar on a daily basis. Adults reported drinking, on average, 28 ounces a day—that's nearly 300 calories—from liquids. Sodas were the main calorie culprits, accounting for 60 percent of the respondents' beverage calories.

Decades ago, beverages provided only 2 to 4 percent of total calories, and today it's about 20 percent of all of our calories.

SLIM SOLUTIONS

MAKE BETTER BEVERAGE CHOICES

Hydrate with water or seltzer before any other beverages. If you drink diet sodas or other diet beverages, limit them, as they drive your desire for additional sweets. Enjoy calorie-free coffee and tea, as they provide beneficial antioxidants, but cut out creamy coffees with fancy toppings (read: caramel and whipped cream!) and teas that can add hundreds of calories.

Skip soda and similar beverages that provide no nutritional benefits other than sugar calories. When you *do* drink beverages, make sure that they're nutrient-rich, like skim milk.

THINK BEFORE YOU DRINK!

In the typical U.S. diet, here's how calories from liquid beverages stack up:

* Soda and sugary drinks: 203 calories
* Alcohol: 99 calories
* Milk: 84 calories
* 100 percent fruit juice: 32 calories
* Coffee/tea: 11 calories

FAT HABIT #78

Beer, wine, sangria . . . bring it on! —EVELYN B.

How can something served in such a little glass or with a pretty little umbrella be so dangerous? As we mentioned above (see Fat Habit #76, "I pig out on weekends!"), alcohol is a true triple threat: It's caloric, it increases appetite, and it lowers inhibitions. If your nights and weekends are filled with social or business commitments, like client dinners, happy hour, and Sunday brunch, you may be adding hundreds of empty alcohol calories.

SLIM SOLUTIONS

Appetite for Health contributor and NYC-based registered dietitian Martha McKittrick shares her tips for putting the brakes on booze:

ID YOUR TROUBLE ZONES

Think about your lifestyle and where potential problem areas might occur. Do you end up sipping more than you planned at happy hour with coworkers? At Sunday brunch with your friends? Keeping a food and alcohol record for a week or two can be very helpful in pinpointing your pitfalls.

TAKE ALCOHOL OUT OF THE EQUATION

Instead of meeting friends for drinks after work, make plans to take a Zumba class or go for a speed walk. You can always grab a healthy dinner afterward, without the alcohol.

SIP SLOWLY

No one will even notice you're still on your first drink as they're getting ready for number three or four. It sounds simple, but it works.

The slower you drink, the less alcohol (and fewer calories) you'll consume. It helps if you order a drink that is meant to be savored, not slurped. "For example, I tend to drink red wine more slowly than white wine. If I wanted to drink really slowly, I'd order a scotch," McKittrick says. Another slow-down strategy: Alternate your glass of wine or drink with a club soda or water.

CUT YOURSELF OFF

Set limits on how many drinks you'll allow yourself each week. Perhaps your goal is five. That means if you want to indulge with your Match.com date and have a few beers at the barbecue, then you'll have to skip drinks with your girlfriends at dinner on Friday night.

ARRIVE FASHIONABLY LATE

When meeting friends for drinks and/or dinner, try to arrive a little late. This way you can skip the martini at the bar before the meal.

GO FOR JOE

Meet dates and friends for coffee instead of drinks.

GIVE YOUR WAITER THE STOP SIGN

Attentive waiters can be trouble—as soon as you turn your head to talk to your dining companion, the waiter is ready to fill your glass. Remain on high alert at parties and subtly cover your glass with your hand so it doesn't get refilled.

MAKE IT A LUNCH DATE

If you have the choice, schedule more of your business meetings around lunchtime. Not too many people drink at lunch these days.

PLAY IT OUT IN YOUR HEAD

Visualize the scenario before heading out to meet your friends. See yourself at the bar saying, "No, thanks," when your pal offers you another drink. Set your goal as to how many drinks you will have before going out, and stay focused throughout the night so you stick to it.

Women and Alcohol: Make That a Double . . . Or Nothing?

We all know that drinking in excess—more than two to three drinks per day for women—isn't a good idea, but what about an occasional drink? Does it help or hurt your health?

Most studies show that alcohol in moderation may offer some benefits, particularly for cardiovascular health. But other research has shown that for some women, even moderate alcohol consumption can raise the risk of breast cancer.

What should you do? Moderate alcohol intake—that's a drink per day for women, two for men—is okay for most healthy people, with a few important caveats:

1. If you or a close relative (a mother, sister, aunt, or grandmother) have a history of breast cancer, you should err on the side of caution and limit/avoid alcohol until more studies are done.
2. Don't start drinking if you don't currently drink just to reap the heart health benefits. There are many other ways to a healthy heart that don't involve drinking. For instance, a diet rich in fruits and vegetables and whole grains can provide important antioxidants and protect your pumper.
3. If you have a history of alcohol addiction, obviously you should avoid alcohol altogether.

FAT HABIT #79

It's the holidays . . . time to gain ten pounds! —Susan V.

Stuffing and eggnog and cookies, oh my! The six weeks from Thanksgiving to New Year's are filled with some of the most calorie-packed foods that we face all year. It's hard for even those with miraculous metabolisms to maintain their weight during this time. Research shows that people who are at a healthy weight gain about a pound during this period.

For those who are overweight or are maintaining a loss, it's even harder. These folks tend to gain about 5 pounds during the holidays. That might not sound too bad, but it's like the gift that keeps on giving, as most people never lose their holiday weight.

SLIM SOLUTIONS

Here's how you can have a healthy holiday season.

DON'T GO HUNGRY

Have a nutritious snack before you hit any holiday party. A 100- to 200-calorie snack containing healthy carbs and protein will help you combat the urge to plow through the buffet table. (See page 213 for top on-the-go snacks.)

LOSE THE BOOZE

For smart sipping strategies, see Fat Habit #78, "Beer, wine, sangria . . . bring it on!"

CHOOSE THE RIGHT COMPANY

Bypass the bunch of ladies at the buffet table and instead keep company with the chatty crew. Your primary objective at holiday parties should be socializing, not eating. Instead of stuffing pastry puffs into your mouth, stay engaged in lively conversation so you can enjoy your evening without suffering the guilt that comes with overeating.

BYOF—BRING YOUR OWN FARE

If you're heading out to a friend's party or an office potluck, consider bringing a low-calorie dish that you know you'll enjoy. You're guaranteed to have at least one item that you know is going to fit your calorie budget.

LIMIT "TASTES" WHEN COOKING

If you do most of the cooking during the holidays, be aware that taste-testing could quickly become an entire meal. Instead of sampling mindlessly every few minutes, limit yourself to two small bites of each item pre- and postseasoning.

WALK IT OFF

Start a new holiday tradition: the family walk. Besides burning some extra calories, it will get everyone away from the food for a while.

FAT HABIT #80

My neighborhood is making me fat. —Jenna B.

The crime rate in your area might be low and you might feel safe walking the streets, but beware: Danger could be lurking on every corner. Those seemingly innocent-looking delis or convenient 7-Elevens are just waiting to lure you in and tempt you.

Don't believe us? Let us take you on a walking tour of some of the Weapons of Mass Diet Destruction in Katherine's neighborhood. Just across the street, the innocently named Corner Café opened last month. They have an incredible array of healthy soups, salads, and sandwiches. It's inexpensive and very convenient. Yet they dedicated an entire counter to enormous cupcakes, pies, brownies, cookies, and almost every sweet delight imaginable. Katherine says, "I go in there with the best of intentions—a mixed-greens salad, plain tuna, extra veggies, and just a bit of balsamic vinaigrette. But it takes significant willpower to get out without buying a five-hundred-plus-calorie belly bomber."

In fact, research shows that even the mere sight of food can trigger unexpected cravings. Sure, you can seek safety in the comfort of your own home, but eventually you're going to have to come out and face the diet dangers lurking in your neighborhood. Here's how to navigate your neighborhood safely:

SLIM SOLUTIONS

GO OUT WITH A GAME PLAN

Don't hit the streets hungry. If you're *really* hungry there's probably no amount of nutrition knowledge, willpower, or tasty salad toppings that can keep you from that beautifully frosted cupcake, if one just happens to glance your way. So don't leave home on an empty stomach.

And to be safe, keep a stash of better-for-you options in your bag. Katherine's favorites: apples, bananas, individually wrapped prunes, small bags of pistachios, and sunflower seeds. (See page 213 for other good on-the-go snacks.)

KEEP A "HEALTHY-ALTERNATIVE" ARSENAL AT HOME

"A lot of times, I'll be able to stave off a 'love-at-first-sight' street-food craving by keeping healthy foods that I like in my kitchen," Katherine says. "For example, if I'm walking back from the gym and I see someone eating a huge, delicious scoop of gelato, I'll go home and have some creamy Greek yogurt instead. No, it's not the same as gelato—I'm not trying to fool anyone here. But it is very tasty and satisfying, and you save about 200 calories versus the gelato."

INDULGE IN MODERATION

Unless it's a food that you know will trigger a binge, it's okay to give in on occasion. In many cases, if you try to completely abstain, it will only backfire. Enjoy a not-so-good-for-you treat once a month, guilt-free.

CHANGE YOUR PATH

Let's face it, sometimes there are foods that you just can't eat in moderation no matter how hard you try. Either they end up as a 2,000-calorie meal or they trigger a binge. If there is a restaurant or food shop in your neighborhood that sells this food, you may need to avoid it altogether. Plan a route that will keep you out of the way of "trigger" shops and restaurants.

FAT HABIT #81

Whenever I hit an all-you-can-eat, I eat all I can. —Josh G.

What is it about buffets that makes us want to stuff ourselves silly: the towering pile of plates, the seemingly limitless number of choices, the pay-one-price fee? All of these may play a role, but don't overlook your thrill-seeking tongue. Scientists have found that an abundance of different flavors at one meal can overstimulate the brain's appetite centers, so you overeat before feeling full.

This tendency to feel full and stop eating when flavors are limited and to do the opposite when flavors are varied is called *sensory-specific satiety.* Research shows that different types of flavors, such as sweet, salty, and sour, activate their own appetite centers in the brain. This explains why you might feel full after eating a savory meal but still have room for dessert, and why the buffet table—or anywhere you're faced with an endless array of foods—can put you into eating overdrive.

SLIM SOLUTION

You can get hold of sensory hunger by remaining conscious of whether you're eating to satisfy your biological hunger or your thrill-seeking tongue.

Ask yourself: "Do I want this food because I am still hungry or am I just interested in its taste?" If you're after a taste, then enjoy a small and mindful bite. (See page 91 for tips on intuitive eating.) You don't have to eat a whole serving just because you're interested in its taste!

Also, cut back on portion sizes to accommodate the sensory-specific satiety. Basically, you're leaving room for the curiosity of your tongue. When faced with a diversity of tastes, choose to taste all you can taste—not necessarily eat all you can eat!

Rethink buffets, potlucks, and other kinds of smorgasbords as gustatory galleries. Peruse; don't abuse.

FAT HABIT #82

I check my luggage, but not my diet, at the airport.
I'm a flying disaster. —Gena T.

As RDs who fly just about every month, we know that airports and flights can present a real nutrition challenge. With increased security measures and flight delays, we're spending more time than ever at the airport. If you don't have a good "flight plan," you may end up killing time by eating a lot of junk, then board your plane and continue eating.

Top-Ranked Healthy-Fareports

Some airports are better than others! Here are the top-ranked "healthier fare" airports in the United States, according to the 2011 report by RDs at the Physicians Committee for Responsible Medicine (PCRM).

1. **Detroit Metropolitan Wayne County Airport.** Detroit tops the list for the third year in a row. It's the only airport in the history of PCRM's report to receive a perfect score—twice. Every restaurant at the airport offers at least one healthful entrée, such as a veggie burrito (hold the cheese) at Diego's Mexican Cantina, the black-bean burger at Slapshotz, and the hummus and veggie platter at the Heineken Lounge.

2. **San Francisco International Airport.** San Francisco lags slightly behind Detroit in second place for the third year. Hungry travelers can enjoy the organic smoky split-pea soup with a hummus and veggie wrap at the San Francisco Soup Company, or a beet salad, tofu wrap, quinoa bowl, or udon noodles at Plant Café and Pinkberry.

3. **Washington Dulles International Airport.** Options for health-conscious passengers include the grilled veggie sandwich (no cheese, please!) at Harry's Tap Room, and pasta with marinara sauce at Famous Famiglia.

4. **Minneapolis–St. Paul International Airport.** Travelers through MSP can enjoy the organic oatmeal or the roasted beet-and-pear salad (hold the cheese) at French Meadow Bakery & Café, or the smoked-tofu burrito or wrap with Cajun, Thai, or teriyaki flavors at 360 Gourmet.

5. **(tie) Dallas/Fort Worth International Airport.** Health-conscious diners can find options including the poblano, potato, and zucchini taco at Urban Taco, and the falafel wrap or three-bean chili at UFood Grill.

5. **(tie) Las Vegas McCarran International Airport.** A smoked-tofu burrito is available at 360 Gourmet, and a vegan wrap with hummus is available at more than ten of the restaurants operated by the HMSHost, including Bar One, Home Turf Sports Bar, and Wipeout Willy's.

6. **(tie) Denver International Airport.** Choices here include the veggie burger at the Boulder Beer Tap House, the portobello mushroom

sandwich at the Colorado Sports Bar, and the Colorado Sunshine Wrap or the tofu wrap at Itza Wrap! Itza Bowl!

6. **(tie) Miami International Airport.** Find yourself waiting at Miami International? Try the hummus platter at Beaudevin, and the unique veggie burger or the Asian veggie salad bowl at the Counter.

7. **(tie) Charlotte Douglas International Airport.** Health-conscious passengers can choose the veggie burger at Stock Car Café and the portobello-mushroom-and-red-pepper sandwich at the Carolina Beer Company.

7. **(tie) Phoenix Sky Harbor International Airport.** Healthier fare at Sky Harbor includes the chopped Mediterranean salad, hummus appetizer, and bruschetta at BarFly, and the veggie rice bowl or burrito (ask for little or no cheese) at Blue Burrito.

8. **Orlando International Airport.** Hungry travelers seeking heart-healthy fare should try the vegetarian lentil chili at McCoy's Bar and Grill, or the vegetarian sandwich at ZaZa's Cuban Café.

9. **(tie) Baltimore/Washington International Airport.** Hanging out at BWI? The Silver Diner remains the best bet for savvy travelers. It offers a portobello vegetarian stir-fry with tofu, veggies, and wheat noodles in teriyaki sauce, as well as a summer salad and a veggie chili with kidney beans, mushrooms, carrots, and squash.

9. **(tie) Los Angeles International Airport.** Healthful highlights include the Vegetarian Works pizza (hold the cheese) at Malibu Al's, vegetable sushi rolls at Sushi Boy, and the roasted-pepper-and-eggplant sandwich at Brioche Dorée.

10. **Ronald Reagan Washington National.** Lighter meals here include the Asian peanut-tofu wrap at Hudson Aero Mart and Hudson Euro Café, or the balsamic garden panini with squash and zucchini (request no cheese).

SLIM SOLUTIONS

GO ONLINE

Before you set foot on the plane, check out the airline's website. Most will have info about in-flight meal options. And with cutbacks, some flights serve no food at all, so be prepared.

BUY BEFORE YOU FLY

If you've had time to bring your own meal from home, congratulations! You've made the best choice . . . and saved some money! (Remember, pack only solid foods, as any liquids won't make it through security.)

But if you're like most of us and running to the airport with few minutes to spare, buying at the airport may be your only option (short of going hungry for hours on end . . . which we definitely don't recommend).

PACK YOUR SNACKS

Especially for shorter flights, you'll be much better off with your own snacks. See our top on-the-go snacks on page 213.

FAT HABIT #83

I always bring home the same souvenir from my vacations . . .
extra pounds! —BARB T.

So you've saved up for a spectacular vacation—even lost a few pounds to look perfect in your swimsuit. But as soon as your plane touches down in your vacation paradise, all your healthy habits go out the window! If you're like most people, here's the math:

Relaxing holiday + heaps of tasty food = an ill-fitting bikini

We're not too crazy about this equation. So here's how we balance vacations with a healthy routine.

SLIM SOLUTIONS

CHOOSE A GOOD SPOT

This seems like a no-brainer, but from a stay-fit perspective, it's important to pick a location where you can get lots of physical activity doing things you *enjoy*! For example, some of my favorite activities include hiking, swimming, and yoga. Katherine says, "When I go on vacation I try to make sure that I'm going to a place where I can do at least one form of exercise every day."

START YOUR DAY OFF RIGHT

A balanced breakfast, like nonfat yogurt with fruit and granola, will fuel morning activity and curb hunger later in the day.

CHOOSE ONE MEAL AS YOUR BIGGER MEAL; MAKE THE OTHER TWO SMALLER

Decide ahead of time what your "splurge" meal will be. Katherine says, "I *love* breakfast. I make that my main 'big' meal when I'm on vacation. It's so easy to overdo it with holiday lunches and dinners, particularly because this often means dining out and larger portion sizes. For lunch I stick with salads (dressing on the side), and for dinner I often share an entrée portion (local seafood is a favorite)."

DO ACTIVITIES YOU *LOVE*

Love hiking and snorkeling? Go for it! Even though you may not feel like you're "working out," anything physical counts. Outdoor activities like biking, hiking, and snorkeling are excellent ways to explore your holiday destination and see things you wouldn't if you just stay in the resort or spa.

FAT HABIT #84

I eat my way through the mall! —KELLIE W.

Somehow shopping and eating seem to go together like, say, peanut butter and chocolate. And it's no wonder! Shopping malls are literally filled to the rafters with tempting smells and quick-serve treats. But buyer beware! Your next shopping spree could push you into a higher dress size if you're not careful.

Just check out this list of Food Court hazzards:

FOOD-COURT FOOD	CALORIES	APPROXIMATE TIME TO SHOP IT OFF*
Cinnabon Caramel Pecanbon	1,080	5 hours
Cinnabon Classic Cinnamon Roll	880	4 hours
Quiznos Small Tuna Melt	750	3 hours, 28 minutes
Auntie Anne's Jumbo Pretzel Dog	610	2 hours, 40 minutes
McDonald's Cheeseburger and Small Fries	550	2 hours, 30 minutes
Jamba Juice Orange Dream Machine	470	2 hours, 5 minutes
Auntie Anne's Cinnamon Sugar Stix	470	2 hours, 5 minutes
Sbarro Cheese Pizza (1 slice)	460	2 hours
Starbucks Blueberry Scone	460	2 hours
Panda Express Mongolian Beef and Veggie Spring Rolls and Sweet and Sour Sauce	440	1 hour, 55 minutes
Quiznos Small Turkey Ranch and Swiss	400	1 hour, 50 minutes
Quiznos Smoky Chipotle Turkey Flatbread Sammie	380	1 hour, 40 minutes
Starbuck Grande Hot Chocolate with Whip	370	1 hour, 40 minutes
Mrs. Fields Double Fudge Brownie	360	1 hour, 40 minutes
Auntie Anne's Original Pretzel	340	1 hour, 30 minutes
Au Bon Pain Asian Chicken Salad w/Half Packet Light Dressing	330	1 hour, 10 minutes

* Based on a 140-pound woman strolling at a leisurely pace

SLIM SOLUTIONS

While the best solution is to avoid food courts at all costs, we realize that's not always possible. In those instances when you must eat and shop, here's how you can make the most of your food-court choices.

Before you hit the mall, eat a filling breakfast of oatmeal, whole-grain cereal, or eggs with whole-grain toast. This will help curb your appetite for several hours.

Once you're there, keep the following tips in mind:

PIZZA POINTERS

If you opt for a slice, ask for thin-crust, as it will help shave calories, and go for veggie-only toppings. If the pie is oozing with cheese, take half of it off before eating.

DOWNSIZE YOUR ORDER

Rather than a main course, order a bowl of soup and a side salad, or two side dishes in place of a main course.

DUMP THE DESSERTS

Little—if anything—can be a calorie bargain among the dessert-type vendors, such as Mrs. Fields, Cinnabon, and ice-cream parlors like Cold Stone Creamery.

LOOK FOR HEALTHY MENU OPTIONS

For example, Panda Express offers Wok Smart menu items that have no more than 250 calories per serving, or order a Subway sandwiche with less than six grams of fat per sandwich (see our fast-food guide on page 186).

SKIP LIQUID CALORIES

Avoid the smoothies and specialty beverages that can have more calories than a fast-food burger. Instead, drink water or seltzer, or have a cup of coffee, tea, or skim latte.

BYOS

Bring your own snacks. Healthy options are those that contain a good amount of fiber to keep you fuller longer. See our "snacks on the go" list on the following page.

SALAD SMARTS

Salads may sound like a good bet, but look at calories before ordering. The dressing can pile on more calories than the entire salad.

Top On-the-Go Snacks

Need healthy snacks you can just pop into your handbag or pick up on the road? Try some of these.

Goat Cheese & Garden Veggies Bistro Box from Starbucks

Laughing Cow Light Cheese Wedges w/ whole-grain crackers

Single-serve pack of Wheat Thins and 1 piece part-skim string cheese

Nutrition bars: Look for bars that contain less than 200 calories, and compare the nutritional labels. Go with the bar that offers more fiber, less sugar, and adequate protein (about 5 to 10 grams). Bars we like: Lärabar, Pure Bar.

Sabra's pretzel-and-hummus combo cups

30 pistachios, 23 almonds, or ¼ cup mixed nuts

¼ cup dry-roasted edamame

¼ cup dried fruit-and-nut mixture

4 to 5 Sunsweet Ones (individually wrapped dried plums)

Planters single-serve trail mix

Apple or banana with "to-go" individual-size peanut butter containers

Hard-boiled egg with 1 slice whole-grain bread.

6-ounce cup Fage, Yoplait Greek, or Chobani non-fat yogurt with ½ banana

2 fig bars

1 apple with 2 tablespoons almond butter

APPETITE FOR HEALTH'S SLIM SOLUTIONS FOURTEEN-DAY MEAL PLAN

FAT HABIT #85

I can't put what I know about healthy eating into practice . . .
as in what to eat for breakfast, lunch, and dinner. —SOPHIE D.

It's four p.m.: Do you know what you're having for dinner? If your answer is something like "I'm still thinking about it," or "I don't have a clue," or "Who should I call for delivery tonight?" your winging-it impromptu approach to meals is probably the most physique-damaging habit of all.

If you need some help organizing what and how much to eat, we can help. We've detailed two weeks of meals and snacks and provide tips for the foods you should be buying at the supermarket. You'll also find extensive lists of dietitian-approved "cheats" so that you don't feel deprived.

Our fourteen-day meal plan incorporates all of the principles that we, and other top nutrition pros, use in our everyday lives. This is where the rubber meets the road: what we cook and eat ourselves.

The focus is on the right portions of quality (read: nutritious!) foods to help you lose weight and learn what you should be eating and how much.

Our meal plan is 100 percent gimmick-free: You can eat real foods from all the food groups, enjoy limited "treats," and still lose weight. We've kept the main meals to 400 calories for a reason: Calories count. The only way to lose weight is to eat fewer calories than you burn off, and by eating about 1,600 calories a day, most women will lose at least a pound a week. In addition, 400 calories is an amount that will help you feel satisfied—but not too much.

By offering three meals of equal calories, we ensure that at least two-thirds of your daily calories are eaten before dinner, which helps the body burn calories more efficiently, keeps hunger at bay, and helps to ensure that what you eat is burned off and not stored as body fat.

EACH DAY'S MEAL PLAN PROVIDES:

- 1,600 calories per day divided between breakfast, lunch, dinner, and two snacks
- Breakfasts, lunches, and dinners that are around 400 calories and provide protein to promote satiety, maintain lean body tissue, and help shift metabolism so that your body burns more fat as fuel
- Mix-and-match meals to suit your taste preferences
- Midmorning and afternoon snacks to keep hunger in check
- 100 "free" calories each day to use on a "treat" food, like sugar or honey in your coffee or tea, half a candy bar, or a small portion of gummy bears.
- Wholesome, natural foods from our core food groups: whole

grains, fruits and vegetables, lean proteins, nonfat and low-fat dairy, and healthy unsaturated fats

- Protein- and/or fiber-rich choices at all meals and snacks to help regulate hunger hormones so you feel fuller on fewer calories
- Our favorite go-to recipes from Chapter 9

THE PLAN LIMITS:

- Nutrient-poor, calorie-rich food and beverages
- Saturated fats and added sugars

CREATE 1,600-CALORIE MEAL PLANS OF YOUR OWN

Use the number of servings and serving sizes listed for each food group to plan your own meals and snacks.

6 SERVINGS GRAINS (PRIMARILY WHOLE GRAINS)

One serving equals about 80 calories.

Suggested serving sizes:

1 ounce breads*: ½ small bagel, 1 slice bread, 1 cup cold cereal,†
  1 light whole-wheat English muffin, ½ hamburger or hot-dog bun, 1 pancake, 1 6-inch pita, ½ 6-inch corn or flour tortilla
½ cup cooked grains: barley, bulgur, rice, oats, quinoa, and pasta
½ cup starchy vegetables like corn, peas, pumpkin
Crackers: 2 sheets (4 squares) graham crackers, 4 pieces melba toast, 20 oyster crackers, 2 saltines

* We recommend breads that contain at least 4 grams protein and 4 grams fiber per slice.
† We recommend cold cereals that provide at least 4 grams protein, 4 grams fiber, and less than 10 grams sugar.

2 FRUIT SERVINGS

One serving equals about 60 calories.

1 medium piece most fruits (apple, orange, 1 small banana or
   ½ medium)
1 cup berries, melon
¼ cup dried fruit
½ cup canned fruit (packed in juice)
6 ounces 100 percent juice

AT LEAST 4 VEGETABLE SERVINGS

One serving equals approximately 25 calories.

1 cup raw or leafy greens
½ cup cooked greens

2 NONFAT OR LOW-FAT DAIRY SERVINGS

One serving equals approximately 80 calories.

1 cup skim milk
1 cup 1 percent milk
1 cup low-fat buttermilk
½ cup evaporated skim milk
⅓ cup dry nonfat milk
6 ounces plain nonfat yogurt
1 cup 2 percent milk
8 ounces plain low-fat yogurt

7 LEAN PROTEIN SERVINGS

One serving equals approximately 55 calories.

BEEF

1 ounce lean beef, such as round, sirloin, and flank steak; tenderloin; or chipped beef

PORK

1 ounce lean pork, such as fresh ham; canned, cured, or boiled ham

VEAL

1 ounce; all cuts are lean except for veal cutlets (ground or cubed)

POULTRY

1 ounce chicken, turkey, Cornish hen (without skin)

FISH

1 ounce fresh and frozen fish

1 ounce crab, lobster, scallops, shrimp, clams (fresh or canned in water)

2 medium canned sardines

CHEESES

½ cup nonfat or low-fat cottage cheese

2 tablespoons grated Parmesan

1 ounce nonfat or low-fat cheese

OTHER

2 egg whites

¼ cup egg substitutes (with fewer than 55 calories per ¼ cup)

4 ounces tofu

5 HEALTHY FATS

One serving equals approximately 45 calories.

1 teaspoon oil (vegetable, corn, canola, olive, etc.)
1 tablespoon reduced-fat margarine or mayonnaise
2 tablespoons reduced-fat or light salad dressing
2 tablespoons light cream cheese
⅛ avocado
8 large black olives

NUTS AND SEEDS
6 dry-roasted almonds
1 tablespoon cashews
2 pecans
20 peanuts (small)
10 peanuts (large)
2 walnuts, whole

FREE FOODS

Enjoy the following foods in moderate amounts:

BEVERAGES
Bouillon, broth, consommé
Club soda
Coffee, unsweetened
Flavored water, carbohydrate-free
Nonfat creamer
Tea, unsweetened
Tonic water, sugar-free
Water: plain, carbonated, mineral

FOODS AND CONDIMENTS

Nonstarchy raw vegetables

Horseradish

Lemon juice

Mustard

Vinegar

Seasonings

Cooking spray

Cooking wine

Flavored extracts: almond, peppermint, vanilla

Garlic

Herbs

Hot pepper sauce

Pimiento

Spices

Worcestershire sauce

GROCERY LIST

Groceries for the meal plan, as well as important healthy staples, are provided in the list below. Remember, having healthy food plays a significant role in weight loss.

FRESH PRODUCE

VEGETABLES

Choose fresh and in-season, whenever possible

Lettuces

Bagged mixed salad greens

Onions

Broccoli

Carrots

Tomatoes

Sweet potatoes/potatoes

Bell peppers

Mushrooms

Cucumbers

Squash

Eggplant

Green beans

FRUIT

Choose fresh and in-season, whenever possible

Avocados

Berries

Citrus (oranges, grapefruit, lemons, limes)

Bananas

Apples

Kiwis

Stone fruits (peaches, nectarines, plums)

Grapes

Melon (watermelon, cantaloupe, honeydew)

Pineapple

FRESH HERBS

Cilantro, garlic, parsley, mint, dill

Gourmet Garden Fresh Blends

DAIRY

Eggs/egg whites

Nonfat plain Greek yogurt

Low-fat cottage cheese

Skim or 1 percent milk

Feta cheese

Parmigiano-Reggiano cheese

Low-fat provolone, Swiss, or Muenster cheese

Babybel Light cheese

Laughing Cow Light Spreadable Wedges

Plain, unsweetened almond milk

Plain, unsweetened soy milk

Light spreadable butter

Soft spread sold in tub

MEAT, POULTRY, SEAFOOD

Turkey or chicken breast

Rotisserie chicken

Ground sirloin or ground bison

Seafood (ideally purchase same day of preparation)

FROZEN FOODS

Light frozen dinners (less than 350 calories and at least 15 grams
protein)

Veggie burgers

Frozen fruit (no added sugar)

Frozen vegetables

Morningstar Farms breakfast patties

PANTRY ITEMS

DRY GOODS/BREADS/GRAINS

Whole-grain, fiber-rich cereals (at least 2 grams fiber, less than
10 grams sugar per serving)

Brown rice, bulgur, quinoa, whole-grain couscous

Whole-grain bread (look for those that have at least 2 grams fiber
and at least 4 grams protein per serving)

Thomas' whole-wheat English muffins or Oroweat whole-wheat or
multigrain Sandwich Thins

Whole-grain pasta

Whole-grain pita pockets

Whole-wheat panko breadcrumbs (e.g., Ian's)

Whole-wheat and all-purpose flour

High-fiber whole-grain cereal bar (look for at least 3 grams fiber
and less than 10 grams sugar per bar)

Small corn and whole-grain tortillas

Whole-grain crackers

NUTS AND BEANS/SOUPS

In-shell pistachios

Walnuts

Almonds

Pine nuts

Flavored nuts, like wasabi-seasoned almonds or Bragg's amino acid
cashews

CONDIMENTS AND CANNED ITEMS

Extra virgin olive oil

Canola oil/sunflower oil

Mustards

Vinegars (balsamic, sherry, champagne)

Hot sauces

Salsa

Ketchup

100 percent fruit spread

Applesauce

Reduced-sodium soy sauce

Maple syrup

Honey
Agave
Canned tomato products
Canned broth-based soups
Canned beans
Olives

DRY HERBS AND SPICES

Basil, black pepper, rosemary, oregano, cinnamon, herbes de Provence, chili pepper, nutmeg, cumin, ginger, cloves, garlic powder, thyme, allspice, bay leaves, caraway seeds, cardamom, cayenne pepper, chives, coriander, curry powder, fennel seed, mustard seed, paprika, red pepper, saffron, sage, tarragon, vanilla.

SNACKS

Baked tortilla chips
Hummus
Bean dip
94 percent fat-free microwave popcorn

BEVERAGES

Seltzer
Tea
Coffee

WEEK ONE

MONDAY

BREAKFAST

1 cup cooked oatmeal with ½ cup nonfat plain Greek yogurt topped
with cinnamon and 1 cup fresh or frozen (no added sugar) berries
Coffee or tea

A.M. SNACK

Snap peas or other fresh veggies with 2 tablespoons hummus

LUNCH

Mediterranean Tuna Salad

1 cup cooked whole-wheat pasta
3 ounces canned light tuna packed in water
6 black olives
2 tablespoons chopped yellow onion
Red bell pepper
Cherry tomatoes
1 ounce feta cheese
2 teaspoons extra virgin olive oil
1 tablespoon champagne or red wine vinegar

▪ Combine all ingredients. Season with fresh-squeezed lemon,
salt, pepper, and fresh parsley.

P.M. SNACK

1 medium apple or small banana with 1½ teaspoons nut butter

DINNER

Muffin-Tin Turkey Meat Loaf (Recipe on page 287)

2 cups tossed salad with 1 ounce shredded low-fat cheese and
1 tablespoon light vinaigrette or store-bought light dressing
Coffee or tea or other calorie-free beverage of choice

TUESDAY

BREAKFAST

Protein Pancakes *(Recipe on page 274)*

With ½ cup nonfat plain Greek yogurt and ½ cup sliced fresh fruit

Coffee or tea

A.M. SNACK

3 or 4 whole-wheat crackers with 1½ teaspoons nut butter

LUNCH

2 ounces sliced turkey deli meat on 2 slices whole-wheat bread with
    lettuce, tomato, mustard, and 2 slices avocado

Fruit salad: 1 cup of any mixed fresh fruit (e.g., berries, grapes,
    apple, melon) topped with chopped fresh mint

Plain or sparkling water with lemon or lime or other calorie-free
    beverage of choice

P.M. SNACK

½ cup nonfat plain Greek yogurt with ¼ cup dried fruit
    (e.g., raisins, cranberries, cherries)

DINNER

1½ cups cooked whole-wheat pasta with ½ cup tomato sauce,
    2 ounces chopped roasted chicken, 1 ounce fresh grated Parmesan cheese, and fresh basil

WEDNESDAY

BREAKFAST

1 cup whole-grain cold cereal or cooked oatmeal with ½ cup skim
    milk or plain nonfat Greek yogurt

1 small banana, sliced, or 1 cup berries

Coffee or tea with ¼ cup nonfat milk or soy milk

A.M. SNACK

8-ounce nonfat or soy latte

LUNCH

Tuna Melt

> *1 whole-wheat English muffin, toasted*
> *3 ounces water-packed tuna (drained) mixed with 1 tablespoon*
> *light mayonnaise and 2 teaspoons pickle relish*
> *1 slice tomato and arugula*
> *1 slice low-fat cheddar cheese*

▪ Layer tuna mixture, tomato, arugula, and cheese on open half of English muffin. Top with other half. Heat in oven until cheese is melted.

Plain or sparkling water with lemon or lime or calorie-free beverage of choice

P.M. SNACK

Veggie crudités with 2 tablespoons light ranch dressing

DINNER

Oven-Fried Chicken Tenders (Recipe on page 293)

2 cups tossed side salad with 1 tablespoon light vinaigrette or reduced-fat dressing

Coffee or tea or other calorie-free beverage of choice

THURSDAY

BREAKFAST

Swiss-Style Muesli (Recipe on page 273) with

1 small banana, sliced

8 ounces nonfat latte or soy latte

A.M. SNACK

2 Laughing Cow Light Creamy Swiss wedges with 3 whole-wheat
crackers

LUNCH

Skinny Cobb Salad

2 cups Romaine or mixed greens
1 hard-boiled egg, sliced
3 ounces cooked chicken breast
½ cup each cherry tomatoes and sliced cucumber
1 tablespoon vinaigrette or reduced-fat dressing

■ Toss ingredients in a bowl. Serve with 1 two-ounce toasted
whole-wheat pita

Plain or sparkling water with lemon or lime or calorie-free beverage
of choice

P.M. SNACK

1 apple with 1½ teaspoon nut butter

DINNER

3 ounces broiled or grilled ground sirloin burger on
1 whole-wheat roll with
lettuce, tomato, mustard, and ketchup

FRIDAY

BREAKFAST

1 package belVita Breakfast Biscuits with 8 ounces nonfat plain
Greek yogurt (or 6-ounce container flavored nonfat Greek
yogurt)
Coffee or tea with ¼ cup skim milk or soy milk

A.M. SNACK

Vegetable crudités with 1 tablespoon reduced-fat ranch dressing for
dipping

8 ounces vegetable juice (low-sodium)

LUNCH

Chicken & Apple Salad

3 ounces cooked, sliced chicken breast
1 medium apple, sliced thin, mixed with
2 cups mixed baby salad greens
1 tablespoon blue cheese
1 tablespoon vinaigrette or reduced-fat dressing

▪ Toss ingredients in a bowl.

Plain or sparkling water with lemon or lime, or calorie-free beverage
of choice

P.M. SNACK

1 cup low-fat cottage cheese with cherry tomatoes

DINNER

3 ounces grilled shrimp with 1 cup cooked wild rice with 2 teaspoons extra virgin olive oil

1 cup grilled asparagus, topped with 1 teaspoon extra virgin olive
oil and fresh squeezed lemon

Coffee or tea with ¼ cup skim milk or soy milk

SATURDAY

BREAKFAST

Open-Faced Egg Sandwich

▪ Spread half of 1 toasted whole-wheat English muffin with
2 teaspoons reduced-fat mayonnaise. Top with arugula, sliced tomato, and 2 soft-boiled eggs.

1 small banana (or equivalent fruit serving)
Coffee or tea with ¼ cup skim milk or soy milk

A.M. SNACK
1 cup nonfat plain Greek yogurt with ¼ cup dried fruit

LUNCH
PB&J Sandwich
■ Spread 1 slice whole-wheat bread with 1 tablespoon peanut butter and 2 teaspoons 100 percent fruit spread. Top with another slice of bread.

1 baked apple (or equivalent fruit serving)

P.M. SNACK
½ cup cottage cheese with 1 cup cubed cantaloupe

DINNER
Swedish Meatballs (Recipe on page 283), served on top of
1 cup cooked egg noodles with 1 teaspoon extra virgin olive oil
2 cups tossed green salad with 1 tablespoon vinaigrette or reduced-
   fat dressing

SUNDAY
BREAKFAST
Spinach, Mushroom, and Leek Frittata (Recipe on page 272)
8 ounces nonfat latte or soy latte

A.M. SNACK
2 fig bars or 1 natural energy bar (i.e., Kind, Lärabar, Pure Bar)

LUNCH
Cranberry-Turkey Panini (Recipe on page 277)
Coffee or tea or other calorie-free beverage of choice

P.M. SNACK

1 cup nonfat plain Greek yogurt mixed with ½ cup sliced
strawberries

DINNER

Baja-Style Fish Tacos *(Recipe on page 276)*

Coffee or tea or other calorie-free beverage of choice

WEEK TWO

MONDAY

BREAKFAST

2 whole-grain waffles, topped with ½ cup nonfat Greek yogurt, 1
small sliced banana, 1 tablespoon chopped walnuts, and 1 tablespoon maple syrup

Coffee or tea with ¼ cup soy or skim milk

A.M. SNACK

Skim café latte or skim cappuccino

½ cup grapes or 1 orange

LUNCH

Fiesta Wrap

▪ Grill 4 ounces chicken and wrap into a whole-grain tortilla with
2 tablespoons salsa, 1 cup fresh greens, and 1 ounce cheddar cheese.

P.M. SNACK

1 cup raw vegetables served with 2 tablespoons hummus

DINNER

Pistachio-Crusted Salmon *(Recipe on Page TK)*

1 cup spinach sautéed in garlic and 1 tablespoon olive oil

Sparkling water with lemon, or calorie-free beverage of your choice

TUESDAY

BREAKFAST

Strawberry-Banana Yogurt Parfait *(Recipe on page 275)*

Coffee or tea with ¼ cup skim milk or soy milk

A.M. SNACK

¼ cantaloupe

½ cup low-fat cottage cheese

LUNCH

Dijon Steak Salad

■ Mix 2 cups leafy greens, 1 cup diced red or yellow peppers, and ½ cup grated carrots with 2 teaspoons olive oil and 1 tablespoon Dijon mustard. Top with 3 ounces cooked sirloin and 1 ounce feta. Serve with 1 small whole-grain roll.

Unsweetened iced tea, sparkling water, or other calorie-free beverage.

P.M. SNACK

1 small whole-wheat pita and 1 cup celery sticks with 3 tablespoons bean dip

DINNER

Orecchiette with Shrimp and Peas

■ Place 3 ounces large cooked shrimp in a pan with 2 teaspoons olive oil, chopped garlic, ½ cup diced tomatoes, and ¼ cup frozen peas. Toss mixture with 1 cup cooked whole-wheat orecchiette and serve with 1 tablespoon grated Parmesan.

Plain or sparkling water or other calorie-free beverage

WEDNESDAY

BREAKFAST

Banana-Almond Butter Toast

▪ Toast 1 slice whole-grain bread and top with 1½ tablespoons almond butter and 1 sliced small banana.

Skim latte with 1 teaspoon sugar

A.M. SNACK

1 mini Babybel light cheese round with 1 cup veggie crudités

LUNCH

Chili-Topped Baked Potato (Recipe on page 279)

Juice spritzer (6 ounces 100 percent fruit juice and mixed with 8 ounces seltzer)

P.M. SNACK

Pistachios (about 30)

DINNER

5 ounces fish fillet
1 cup fresh steamed broccoli
1 cup brown rice

▪ Bake or broil a 5-ounce fish fillet with 2 teaspoons olive oil, lemon juice, and seasonings.

Plain or sparkling water or other calorie-free beverage

THURSDAY

BREAKFAST

1 cup cooked oatmeal or oat bran with ½ cup skim milk
¼ cup raisins
Coffee or tea with ¼ cup nonfat milk or soy milk

A.M. SNACK

1 medium pear with 1½ teaspoons almond butter

LUNCH

Spinach-Feta Stuffed Pita

▪ In a small bowl, combine 2 cups chopped raw spinach, 1 cup diced tomato, 2 tablespoons crumbled feta cheese, and 2 tablespoons low-fat cream cheese. Stuff the mixture into 1 small whole-wheat pita and heat or microwave until cheese is melted.

Iced tea or other calorie-free beverage

P.M. SNACK

2 ak-mak crackers or whole-grain crackers
1 ounce low-fat cheese

DINNER

Mexican Quinoa and Black Bean Salad *(Recipe on page 292)*
Plain or sparkling water with lemon or lime

FRIDAY

BREAKFAST

Breakfast Patty Sandwich

▪ Layer 1 cooked soy patty and 1 slice 2 percent American cheese between 2 whole-wheat English muffin halves.

Skim café latte with 1 teaspoon sugar

A.M. SNACK

1 cup veggies with ¼ cup bean dip

LUNCH

Shrimp, Feta, and Couscous *(Recipe on page 293)*

100 percent fruit juice spritzer (6 ounces 100 percent fruit juice and 8 ounces seltzer)

P.M. SNACK

1 sliced tomato drizzled with 2 teaspoons olive oil and seasonings

DINNER

Beef Brisket with Asparagus

- Coat 12 asparagus spears with 1¼ teaspoons olive oil and grill until tender.
- Serve with 1 cup cooked brown rice and 3 ounces precooked lean beef brisket.

SATURDAY

BREAKFAST

Egg-White Scramble

- Scramble 4 egg whites with 1 slice low-fat cheese and 1 cup diced tomato.
- Serve with 1 slice whole-wheat toast spread with 2 teaspoons trans fat–free margarine and ½ grapefruit.

Skim latte

A.M. SNACK

2 graham crackers spread with 2 tablespoons light cream cheese

LUNCH

Salmon Melt Florentine (Recipe on page 278)
2 cups mixed greens and 1 tablespoon vinaigrette
Plain or sparkling water with lemon or lime

P.M. SNACK

1 cup blueberries with 2 tablespoons light whipped topping

DINNER

Stir-Fry Chicken

▪ Cook 4 ounces skinless chicken breast until center is no longer pink (cut into strips) in 2 teaspoons extra virgin olive oil. Stir in 1 cup mixed vegetables and 2 teaspoons low-sodium soy sauce.

▪ Serve with 1 cup whole-wheat couscous.

SUNDAY

BREAKFAST

1 cup nonfat plain Greek yogurt
1 cup whole-grain cereal with ½ cup skim or soy milk
1 cup strawberries
½ tablespoon chopped walnuts
Unsweetened tea or coffee with skim milk

A.M. SNACK

¼ cup roasted soy nuts

LUNCH

Roast Beef Wrap (Recipe on page 282)

2 cups mixed greens and 1 tablespoon vinaigrette
Unsweetened iced tea or plain or sparkling water with lemon or lime

P.M. SNACK

Skim latte or cappuccino

DINNER

1 turkey patty (150–160 calories) with 1 slice low-fat cheese on whole-grain bun, topped with lettuce and tomato
1 cup steamed broccoli
Calorie-free beverage

FAT HABIT #86

If I cheat on a diet, I feel like a failure and then just give up.

—JOELLE A.

Living lean for life means you're going to slip up. You may totally pig out for a day, a week, or maybe even a month. However, that still doesn't mean you should throw in the towel. Remember: progress, not perfection.

SLIM SOLUTION

One of the more effective ways to guarantee diet success is to build little "treats," or foods you just can't live without, into your meals and snacks. We're like everyone else: Julie needs a little gummy candy in her life, and Katherine enjoys frozen yogurt.

Here's how this can help you. Each day, you have about 120 calories that you can use on whatever you want, as long as you don't go over that limit. If you love potato chips, eat up to 120 calories' worth of them (that's about 20 chips, depending upon the brand). If chocolate is more your thing, 120 calories is about ½ to ¾ ounce of most milk and dark chocolate.

Enjoy up to 120 calories of sweets, savory treats, or candy (calories may vary outside the 80–120 calorie range where noted).

80–120 CALORIES OF TREATS

1 ounce angel food cake with ½ cup sliced strawberries

1 Reese's peanut butter cup

½ to ¾ ounces milk or dark chocolate (check label)

3 pieces hard candy

1 frozen fruit Popsicle

½ cup light ice cream or frozen yogurt

1 tablespoon chocolate syrup

1 tablespoon jam

2 tablespoons light pancake syrup

1½ tablespoons honey or agave

30 plain M&M's

2 tablespoons (7 to 9) peanut M&M's

14 gummy bears

4 to 5 chocolate malt balls

7 gumdrops

6 ounces soda or sweetened beverage

1 chocolate 100-calorie Vita Top or VitaBrownie

6 ounces Yoplait light yogurt

1 Weight Watchers dark chocolate raspberry ice cream bar

4 ounces Mott's applesauce with 1 tablespoon chopped walnuts

½ cup sorbet

16 popchips!

12 hard pretzel sticks

15 Guiltless Gourmet tortilla chips

4 Hershey's milk chocolate Kisses

4 teaspoons mini semisweet chocolate chips

5 cups 94 percent fat-free microwave popcorn

25 Jelly Belly jelly beans

45 mini marshmallows

27 Reese's Pieces

8-ounce hot chocolate packet (made with water)

6 Ritz Bitz—peanut butter flavor

15 Cheez-It crackers

1 100-calorie pouch Goldfish (or about 25 pieces)

2 Pepperidge Farm Milano cookies

1 Nonni's toffee-almond biscotti

2 Lu Pim's orange cookies

2 Keebler Fudge Stripes cookies

3 bite-size Famous Amos chocolate-chip cookies

2 Chips Ahoy! chewy chocolate-chip cookies

5 Keebler Vanilla Wafers

6 Nilla wafers

2 Oreo cookies

10 Junior Mints

10 Pringles original crisps

2 Snickers minis

4 Rolos

1 Fun Size Milky Way bar

8 Milk Duds

5 large Swedish fish

1 Tofutti Cutie (130 calories)

1 Edy's strawberry fruit bar

1 Skinny Cow Mmmmocha Truffle Bar

1 100-calorie Klondike bar

¼ cup Kozy Shack no-sugar-added chocolate pudding (70 calories)

Alcohol: Alcohol is limited to no more than two drinks per week, which count as the 100 discretionary (aka "treat") calories. We recommend abstaining when you're losing weight, but we also know that it's not always realistic for everyone. A serving of alcohol equals 4 ounces wine, 1 ounce distilled spirits, or 12 ounces light beer.

STRONG IS THE NEW SKINNY

DID YOU LOSE YOUR MOTIVATION TO MOVE SOMEWHERE BETWEEN the piles of laundry that need to get done and the fifty-hour-a-week job you're holding down? Like many women, do you feel too time-crunched to do a crunch? Does cutting calories seem a lot easier than sweat-dripping-hard workouts?

Most part-time exercisers find a lot of reasons for not working up a sweat: "It's boring," "The class doesn't fit my schedule," or "That's too hard for me." As a result, 60 percent of us don't meet the minimum guidelines for physical fitness, and a full one-quarter are out-and-out couch potatoes.

We're here to change all of that. We've got a Slim Solution to help you break through your exercise inertia to get you going, and to keep you motivated to continue to move. Like any habit, it requires work at first, but then once it's a habit, you'll wonder how you ever lived without a daily dose of fitness in your life.

FAT HABIT #87

I'm too time-crunched to even think about a crunch. —SUSAN S.

Lack of time is the number-one reason adults cite when asked why they don't work out. The American College of Sports Medicine recommends 150 minutes of moderate-intensity exercise each week, while the Institute of Medicine (IOM) recommends roughly twice as much, or sixty minutes per day.

If you think thirty minutes is *waaay* too much of a time commitment, the good news is that you can break the thirty minutes into three ten-minute sessions. But any amount of exercise is always better than being sedentary. As long as you're gradually doing more than you're now doing, you're making progress. And as we've said before, we advocate progress, not perfection.

We've found that a great alternative to longer, moderate-intensity exercise for those with less time is to focus on short, higher-intensity workouts.

SLIM SOLUTIONS

For some perspective, if you're one of those adults who are inactive some 3,900 minutes each week, you should keep in mind that 150 minutes of exercise equals just 3.8 percent of that time. Hopefully you'll see more opportunities to squeeze several ten- or fifteen-minute sessions into your day.

New research suggests that breaking workouts into shorter sessions (as little as ten minutes) can boost your metabolism, improve your cardiovascular endurance, and help burn extra calories. Start by doing one or two ten-minute sessions a day and try to work up to three (see Fat Habit #89, "I have only ten minutes to spare," for more ideas). If you watch one hour of TV, you get nearly twenty

---

Exercise by Numbers

- More than 60 percent of adults do not achieve the American College of Sports Medicine's exercise guidelines.
- 25 percent of all adults are inactive.
- 60 percent of Americans' awake time—about sixty-five hours a week—is spent being sedentary.
- Americans spend, on average, four and a half hours watching TV every day.
- An estimated 250,000 premature deaths in the United States annually are directly attributable to physical inactivity.
- Physical inactivity is considered as harmful as smoking.

---

minutes' worth of commercials, and you can do these exercises during the commercials.

TEN-MINUTE AEROBIC WORKOUT

Whether you like to walk, run, or bike, here's a proven way to boost your fitness fast. Alternate between high-intensity, one-minute intervals of your activity (a perceived exertion score of 7 out of 10, with 10 being your maximal exertion) followed by a minute of rest; repeat ten times.

FIFTEEN-MINUTE CIRCUIT WORKOUT

This workout combines strength training and aerobic conditioning. Walk or jog at a brisk pace for two minutes; then stop and perform each of the following five exercises between two-minute walk/jogs:

1. | *Push-ups and Air Squats (thirty seconds of each).* To do an air squat, stand with your feet shoulder-width apart, with toes pointed slightly outward. Tighten your abdominal muscles and

push your butt and hips back first, then down, like you're sitting in a chair. Keep your upper body as upright as possible (avoid bending forward at your waist) and your weight in your heels. Lower yourself until your thighs are parallel to the ground (or slightly below). As you lower your body, raise your arms up and in front of your torso to counterbalance your weight; return to starting position.

2. | *Walking Lunges*

3. | *Sit-ups*

4. | *Mountain Climbers.* Begin in a push-up position on the hands and toes. Bring the right knee in toward the chest, resting the foot on the floor. Jump up and switch feet in the air, bringing the left foot in and the right foot back. You can also run the knees in and out rather than touching the toes to the floor. Continue alternating feet as fast as you can for sixty seconds.

5. | *Burpees.* Begin in the standing position; then do a squat and put your hands on the floor in front of you. Then kick your feet behind you so you're in a push-up position. Lower your chest to the ground like you're in a push-up position and pull your feet back into squat position, and then end in full extended standing position with a jump in the air while clapping overhead.

FAT HABIT #88

If I'm healthy, it really doesn't matter whether I exercise. —CASEY L.

Not really . . . would you consider smoking cigarettes to be okay?

Physical activity can help prevent and treat some forty different chronic diseases, from heart disease and certain cancers to type 2 diabetes and osteoporosis. A recent report published in the *Lancet* reported that physical inactivity accounts for some 6 to 10 percent of all preventable deaths. That makes a couch-potato lifestyle as unhealthy as smoking.

You probably wouldn't consider smoking ("I don't want to get cancer!"), but a lazy lifestyle is as bad for your health, and also boosts your risk for cancer. A recent study published in the journal *Cancer* found that women who had the greatest amount of moderate activity in their lives experienced a 30 percent reduction in risk for breast cancer. Making sure you get more physical activity is one of the best ways to help manage your weight (especially after successfully losing weight), and it will improve your overall quality of life. We think you deserve that!

SLIM SOLUTION

Evaluate how you spend your free time; if you're spending more than two hours a day in front of your TV, chances are your muscles and mind are craving more movement.

If you're active during the day (e.g., you stand for work, you're chasing after kids all day, or you have a job that requires you to be physical), then you probably do get more exercise than the average person, and just adding a few structured strength- and flexibility-specific movements will help improve your health and muscle tone.

Review the American College of Sports Medicine's Physical Activity Guidelines (see Fat Habit #92, "I don't lift weights") and see whether you're meeting these guidelines. If you're not yet meeting them, develop a plan to start improving your fitness—and health.

FAT HABIT #89

I have only ten minutes to spare . . . that won't do any good.

—HEATHER J.

The recommended exercise guidelines are a lot for many people to accomplish, but a growing number of time-pressed individuals are finding their way to fitness with short, ten-minute bouts of exercise. Sure, you won't develop the aerobic endurance to run a marathon or complete a triathlon, but you can get yourself fitter in as little as ten minutes.

SLIM SOLUTIONS

The key is to use ten minutes a day to do high-intensity, total-body conditioning. We'll take a page from the CrossFit-style workouts to accomplish this. Here are three ten-minute workouts. You'll be surprised how much fitter you'll get by doing these every day. Build up a repertoire of ten to twenty different ten-minute workouts that focus on various movements for the best results.

WORKOUT 1: RUN PLUS TEN-MINUTE WORKOUT
Run for a minute and, at each minute, stop and do the following exercises:

Minute 1: push-ups
Minute 2: sit-ups
Minute 3: walking lunges
Minute 4: air squats
Minute 5: burpees

WORKOUT 2: TEN-MINUTE CROSS-FIT AMRAP
Doing an AMRAP (as many repetitions as possible) means completing as many rounds as possible in ten minutes. You'll want to go all-out and do as many reps of each movement as you can. You can repeat this WOD (workout of the day) every few weeks to see whether you are getting through more rounds and reps in the ten minutes.

The exercises are as follows:

5 burpees
10 air squats
15 push-ups
20 sit-ups

WORKOUT 3

2 minutes max repetitions of push-ups
Rest 1 minute
2 minutes max repetitions of sit-ups
Rest 1 minute
2 minutes max repetitions of air squats
Rest 1 minute
1 minute max repetitions of burpees

There are numerous websites devoted to CrossFit travel WODs. These WODs generally require no special equipment and are usually anywhere from five to fifteen minutes in length. They're never boring and will be over before you know it.

Here are a couple of websites:

The Traveling WOD: www.thetravelingwod.com/p/traveling-wods
.html
100 Travel CrossFit Workouts: www.crossfitsteelecreek.com/about/
the-workouts/100-travel-workouts

FAT HABIT #90

*I'm too self-conscious to work out. . . . I don't even
know what I'd wear.* —TARA P.

There are so many body-conscious women (and men) who can't get the nerve to start exercising because of internal fears and insecurities that they struggle with. One client told us she was terrified to go into her local gym for fear of sticking out or being the butt of jokes. She would drive to the gym and sit in the parking lot, where she'd proceed to talk herself out of going in.

Others tell us that they don't have anything to wear to work out, or there is no way they're wearing spandex or way-too-revealing athletic apparel, and others just don't want anyone watching them.

The good news is that many, many others before you were in the same boat, so we have lots of great tricks for how these formerly fitness-shy individuals overcame their fears.

SLIM SOLUTION

We get it. Everyone is at least a little self-conscious. But at some point, you need to realize that your own insecurities are keeping you from reaching your health, fitness, and weight-loss goals.

Trust us: If you just try something, you'll feel more self-assured and more confident. You'll feel worse by not doing something than if you actually try a workout. Our client who'd sit in her car in the gym's parking lot and talk herself out of working out hated herself when she did that. Decide that you deserve to improve your health and fitness, and that you have to care less about what others may think and care and more about how you're hurting yourself.

BOTTOM LINE: JUST DO IT!

5 WAYS TO OVERCOME FITNESS SHYNESS

1. | Overcome your apparel dilemmas by simply wearing anything that feels comfortable. If that is a baggy T-shirt and sweatpants, that's great. As long as you have something to wear that allows you to comfortably move, put it on and go for it. You don't have to wear anything that's tight to get fit; nor do you need specific workout clothes. A good pair of shoes is about all you need.

2. | Begin an at-home workout program by purchasing some DVDs, or just put your computer in an area where you can follow some of the exercise videos available on YouTube.

3. | Hire a personal trainer or coach. One of the best ways to feel more secure about working out is having instruction from an expert.

4. | Find a women's-only gym. Gyms for women only are widely available, and most yoga studios have classes that are usually all women. Often, being with a group of women makes a newbie feel more comfortable.

5. | Exercise in off-peak hours. Exercising in the early morning, going to the gym at midday, or walking in the evening makes you less likely to run into crowds. Once you gain some confidence, you'll want others around to see your progress.

FAT HABIT #91

I'm bored with exercise . . . and I never see any results for my hard work. —BECKY D.

If you find exercise boring, we'll assume that you're not participating in something you love, or you've been doing the same thing for months, years, or even, in some cases, decades. Yawn! That even sounds boring.

Julie can totally relate to this, and says she suffers from "exercise ADD," so she needs constant variety to avoid boredom. After years of endurance training, she started CrossFit training to add to her endurance workouts. CrossFit is based on short, high-intensity interval-training workouts that combine elements of strength training, gymnastics, and aerobic conditioning. The workouts are so varied that it may take six months to a year before you actually repeat one. That's how she keeps her workouts fresh and avoids boredom.

Trying something different not only will give you a fresh perspective but also will help you see results. Our bodies adapt to exercise in a matter of weeks, so if we aren't constantly changing the type of movement, intensity, or duration, we will plateau—just as with a weight-loss plateau, you'll experience an exercise plateau. To get real results from exercise, you need to constantly challenge or stress your muscles, which can be from doing different types of sports, working at higher intensities (e.g., interval training, hills), or increasing the time spent during each session. For the best results, you should change your routine every four to five weeks, and you should include some cardio exercise along with strength and flexibility training in your program.

SLIM SOLUTION

The beauty of physical activity and getting fit is that it never should be boring, because you can always find some type of activity you enjoy, and you should be changing it up frequently so that you always have something new and exciting to focus on. Sometimes it may be what you are doing for exercise or at the gym that you find boring, and getting more creative about how you get in shape will solve your problem.

There are so many choices for aerobic exercise (swimming, biking, running, walking, hiking, rowing) and myriad strength-training options (videos, gyms, CrossFit, boot camps, resistance bands, body weight, Pilates), you can find something that's fun and exciting to you.

Here's how to take "boring" out of your workout vocabulary:

- The word "exercise" sounds like work, so banish that word from your vocabulary. Call it your playtime, your daily activity, whatever. Just don't call it exercise.

- Working out is not punishment, so do what you enjoy. If hikes and bike rides aren't your thing, don't do them. There's nothing worse than trying to will yourself to do something you just don't want to do.

- Sign up for an athletic event. There's nothing like signing up for a 10K, marathon, century bike ride, or major mountain climb to get you in shape. Just knowing in the back of your mind that you have the event will keep you honest to your workouts.

- Get a training plan online or from a coach and stick to it. Sometimes when you have a goal or purpose to your workouts, they go by a lot quicker and you'll enjoy them more.

- Buy a cute workout top, bottoms, or awesome sneakers, and allow yourself to wear it only when you're enjoying your new "me time."

- Get some friends to take a class with you. Ask some of the people around you whom you like to socialize with whether they'd be interested in taking a local kickboxing, Spin, CrossFit, or some other type of class. Sweating can be fun—when your friend is with you.

- If you get bored with the cardio equipment at the gym, set mini goals of lasting for just ten to fifteen minutes on four different machines, like the treadmill, elliptical, Spin bike, and indoor rowing machine. Have a specific workout in mind for each of them, and just get through those ten to fifteen minutes; then move on to the next one.

- Break longer cardio workouts into manageable nuggets of work. (See Fat Habit #89, "I have only ten minutes to spare," for ten-minute solutions.)

FAT HABIT #92

I don't lift weights because I don't want to look like a man.

—HEATHER K.

We hear this all the time, and nothing could be farther from the truth. If you've shied away from weights for fear that you're going to look like a bodybuilder, you have nothing to worry about . . . unless you're taking growth hormones or steroids.

Women naturally have much lower levels of testosterone and other "muscle-building" hormones than men do, so even when we lift heavy weights or spend hours working out, we just don't bulk up like guys do.

Strength training is proving to be increasingly important for weight loss. Sure, you burn more calories per minute doing cardio, but without strength training, you won't have the muscle tone that you'll want to keep your body's engine revving like a Porsche, not a Prius. When you gain lean muscle, you'll boost your metabolism, because muscle burns hotter than fat tissue.

Having more muscles also helps you reduce in size. Because muscle mass is so compact, you can have more of it and actually fit into smaller clothes than when you have more body fat.

Most important, having muscle mass can help you turn back the clock, as we lose muscle mass with each passing year after about age 35. It also helps us prevent injury and maintain the functional strength needed to live independently as we age.

Do you really want to be the elderly lady in the ads screaming, "Help! I've fallen and I can't get up"? Really? Julie reminds herself of that every time she does burpees and is pushing herself up off the floor. She swears she never wants to be *that* lady.

SLIM SOLUTION

We believe strong is the new skinny, and that a strong body is a healthy body. To get a stronger, leaner physique, we recommend following the American College of Sports Medicine guidelines, and strength-training two or three times a week (see the following page). We suggest making the most out of each session by doing eight different exercises that target the major muscles of your body—glutes/hamstrings, abs/core, quads, shoulders, back, and arms.

You can use your body weight for many exercises, or go to a gym and use free weights or machines. Free weights are superior, because they require more core muscle engagement to balance muscles and move the weight through the entire range of motion. Be sure to mix up your exercises frequently to continually challenge your muscles for the most benefits. There are so many ways to work your major muscle groups that we'll list just a few options for each:

Glutes/hamstrings: squats, dead lifts, step-ups onto box, lunges, leg curls
Abs/core: crunches, reverse crunches, planks, side planks, leg raises
Chest: bench presses, dumbbell flys, push-ups
Quadriceps: squats, lunges, leg extensions, leg presses
Shoulder: overhead presses, lateral and front raises, push-ups
Back: back extensions, one-armed rows, lat pull-downs
Biceps: curls, push-ups
Triceps: triceps extensions, triceps dips or kickbacks, push-ups

AMERICAN COLLEGE OF SPORTS MEDICINE
PHYSICAL ACTIVITY GUIDELINES

CARDIOVASCULAR EXERCISE

- Get at least 2⅓ hours of moderate-intensity exercise per week.
- Exercise recommendations can be met through 30–60 minutes of moderate-intensity exercise (five days per week) or 20–60 minutes of vigorous-intensity exercise (three days per week).
- One continuous session and multiple shorter sessions (of at least 10 minutes) are both acceptable to accumulate desired amount of daily exercise.
- Gradual progression of exercise time, frequency, and intensity is recommended for best adherence and least injury risk.
- People unable to meet these minimums can still benefit from any amount of activity.

RESISTANCE TRAINING

- Two to four sets of each exercise will help improve strength and power.
- For each exercise, 8–12 repetitions improve strength and power, and 15–20 repetitions improve muscular endurance.

FLEXIBILITY

- Do flexibility exercises at least two or three days each week to improve range of motion.
- Each stretch should be held for 10–30 seconds to the point of tightness or slight discomfort.
- Repeat each stretch two to four times, accumulating 60 seconds per stretch.
- All types of stretching are effective.
- Flexibility exercise is most effective when the muscle is warm. Try light aerobic activity or a hot bath to warm the muscles before stretching.

NEUROMOTOR TRAINING

- Neuromotor exercise (sometimes called "functional fitness training") is recommended for two or three days per week.
- Exercises should involve motor skills (balance, agility, coordination, and gait), proprioceptive exercise training and multifaceted activities (i.e., CrossFit, yoga, Pilates).
- 20–30 minutes per day is appropriate for neuromotor exercise.

FAT HABIT #93

My personal trainer keeps telling me what I should be eating.

—FRANCES K.

Personal trainers, coaches, and yoga instructors are notorious for giving diet advice. While trainers and instructors often have awesome physiques, it doesn't mean that they provide smart diet advice. Most fitness professionals have no educational background in nutrition or weight management, so their knowledge may come from the "school of hard knocks" rather than accredited universities.

Just because your trainer follows a paleo diet, has sworn off dairy products, and believes fruit shouldn't be eaten before noon, doesn't mean that it's right or that you should heed his advice. We've heard countless stories of what trainers have told clients to eat (and not eat), and it can be downright shocking. In some cases, it may even be harmful to your health and well-being.

Trainers are generally working out several hours a day—unlike most of us, who sit on our butts for hours on end every day—so their tight, toned muscles are more from their activities and not their diet. Believe us: Stick with your trainer for exercise advice, and when it comes to what and how much to eat, look for a nutrition professional.

SLIM SOLUTION

Trainers and coaches also know that the results you want to get (like losing inches or seeing some definition in your abs) are 80 percent diet and 20 percent fitness-related. They understand that if they can get you, their client, to eat a diet that results in weight loss, you'll be happier with your fitness results.

If you have a trainer who's feeding you questionable nutrition information, you need to bring a dose of skepticism with you to your workouts. You can simply tell her that you've found some professional registered dietitians that you're now working with to improve your diet. When she tries to encourage you to try a new product or approach to eating, you can also ask her to bring in the peer-reviewed research to back up what she's recommending.

We've found that the more firmly you disengage with trainers about diet and nutrition advice, the more they eventually get it and stick to what they know best—training—and let the nutrition professionals handle nutrition and diet advice.

FAT HABIT #94

I really only care about how my abs look. I'm going to do two hundred sit-ups a night. —ORIANNA T.

"Fab abs," "Flat-belly diet," "Hard abs made easy," "How to get a six-pack."

Headlines like these are everywhere. In fact, there are more than 500 million Google hits for "ab articles." Oodles of websites and blogs are devoted entirely to our "abspirations."

As a nation, we're clearly ab-sessed! In fact, surveys show that about two-thirds of us say that the body part we want to improve upon most is our—you guessed it—abs. Women do more exercises to strengthen their abs than any other muscle group, yet few are seeing any results. What's the real flat-belly secret?

SLIM SOLUTION

A six-pack is not created by crunches, planks, V-sits, side bends, wood choppers, or any other ab-specific exercise, because the exercises don't burn enough calories to help you lose body fat.

People who can't see definition in their midsection have too much body fat that's covering their rectus and transverse abdominis and internal and external obliques. So even if you did a thousand crunches every night, you would not really see any definition in your midsection, unless you dieted too.

Most women will begin to see some ab definition when their body fat is less than 18 percent—but the average American woman is at about 30 percent body fat. Elite athletes and fitness models you see attached to the "fab ab" articles have about 12 to 15 percent body fat.

To get to the abs of your dreams, focus on the menu plan and diet provided in Chapter 7, and don't skip the cardio exercise that

Five Red Flags of Bad Diet Advice

- Requires buying special foods or supplements
- Eliminates entire food groups, like no dairy products or grains
- Promises a quick fix or rapid weight loss (more than 2 to 3 pounds per week)
- Relies on personal anecdotes rather than peer-reviewed science
- Sounds too good to be true

For more ways to recognize bad nutrition advice, see Fat Habit #28, "I try all the latest diets and nothing seems to work."

helps you burn calories. In addition, focusing on strengthening all of your major muscles with strength training will also help you reach your goals.

FAT HABIT #95

Ugh! I can't motivate to get going. . . . I keep saying I'll do it tomorrow. Today is yesterday's tomorrow and I've done nothing.

—MOLLY P.

A body in motion tends to stay in motion and a body at rest tends to stay at rest. —NEWTON'S FIRST LAW OF MOTION

When your giddyap-'n'-go has gotten up and left, it's hard to muster the motivation to move. Lack of motivation is one of the top reasons adults cite in surveys for why they don't exercise. Exercise inertia (also called exercise resistance) is one of the hardest things to combat to get on a workout routine. The first day is the worst, and then it gets easier.

Most of us suffer from some degree of exercise resistance, including many of the top athletes in the world. The good news is that because many of us suffer from the natural tendency to remain at rest, there are all kinds of tools available to get you back on the exercise track. And there's more good news: Once your body is in motion, it's easier to keep it in motion. To get you over the hump, here's what you can do.

SLIM SOLUTIONS

BEAT EXERCISE INERTIA

Think about all the reasons you don't want to exercise and what's stopping you from starting. Then begin answering these questions:

What do I want out of exercise? Write down five to ten things you want from moving your body. For example: "I want to tone up and slim down; boost my energy; fit into my clothes better; run a 5 or 10K."

What's stopping me? Once you've written down what you want from becoming active, now write down your perceived barriers. This could be a physical limitation, like a bad back or knee, or a lack of time, lack of money for the gym, feeling too out of shape, etc.

SET FITNESS GOALS

Now, with your pen in hand, write one or two specific, measurable, achievable goals.

Your goal needs to have a start and finish and must be measurable. An example: "I will walk at least thirty minutes a day, three days a week for the next month."

PSYCH YOURSELF UP, NOT OUT

Negative thoughts about healthy behaviors often stop us from reaching our goals. If you constantly think, "Healthy food tastes bad," you won't want to eat good-for-you choices. The same is true with fitness. If you're telling yourself, "I hate this workout," you will really start to feel that way.

Instead, focus on some positive affirmations:

I feel great when I'm _____ (running, cycling, swimming—fill in the blank).
I love how _____ makes me feel.
I can't wait to _____ today.
_____ will make me smile today.
_____ will give me more energy to get through my day.
_____ will make me feel so accomplished today.

WRITE IT DOWN

Just like we recommend a diet journal, we also recommend an exercise journal so you can see your progress and help yourself overcome your aversion to exercise. Use your journal or online tracker to monitor your progress, and have a reward when you reach your goal.

TRY THE TEN-MINUTE RULE

As Woody Allen said, "Half of life is just showing up." Half of getting on board with fitness is just showing up. Tell yourself, "I have to do this for only ten minutes." Once ten minutes are over, you can stop.

HAVE A BACKUP PLAN

For the days when you just don't want to do anything, have a backup plan, like a yoga class or an exercise DVD that you can do.

CALL A FRIEND

Get on the phone and call up a friend to meet you. That way you'll have the added pressure of letting someone else down if you're a no-show.

USE HOUSECLEANING AS MISSED-WORKOUT PUNISHMENT

If you skip a workout, make yourself spend the same amount of time you would have with your workout doing heavy cleaning at home. Do the laundry; make beds; clean the kitchen or bathrooms. Julie will do almost any exercise to get out of cleaning bathrooms!

FAT HABIT #96

I exercise, so I can eat whatever I want. —ROBIN R.

We wish this were true . . . especially Julie, who has been an athlete her entire life and has learned the hard way that there's nothing farther from the truth. This Fat Habit is particularly common among endurance athletes, who spend hours and hours every day training.

A recent study found that 11 percent of those training for a marathon had no changes in body weight, and 11 percent gained weight! I don't know about you, but I'd think many marathoners expect to lose weight with the amount of training required to finish the 26.2-mile race.

When compared with the ginormous number of calories we can eat, say, in a fast-food meal, a chocolaty brownie, or a plate of pasta, even the most exhaustive exercise can't make much of a dent to help us lose weight.

SLIM SOLUTION

If you need to run an hour just to burn off your a.m. Frappuccino, or walk more than two hours to burn off a Pizza Hut serving of cheese pizza, you'll quickly realize that your exercise can never keep up with an out-of-control diet. To lose weight and get into great shape, you need a healthy, calorie-controlled diet and exercise.

Many active women find that exercise boosts their appetite so much that it's hard to eat less to lose weight. Others eat the same quantity of food every day, regardless of whether they're working out or having a rest day, which makes losing weight nearly impossible.

Here's how to make your workouts work for you, not against you, when trying to lose weight.

Five Ways to Avoid Athletes' Diet Mistakes

BALANCE CALORIES IN WITH CALORIES OUT

We've established that you can't eat whatever you want, even if you're training for a marathon or triathlon. However, when you have big training days you can eat more, but on days that you aren't exercising, eat less. If you're hungry, manage your hunger with our satisfying meal plans and recipes (Chapters 7 and 9).

DIET AT NIGHT

"To have energy to fuel your workouts, eat the majority of your calories earlier in the day and diet at night. Going to bed slightly hungry is a lot easier than trying to work out when you feel like there's nothing in the tank." —Nancy Clark, MS, RD, CSSD (www.nancyclarkrd.com), author of *Food Guide for Marathoners: Tips for Everyday Champions*

STOP WISHFUL THINKING

"Don't think, 'I just finished a great workout; now I can eat whatever I want!' This type of thinking gets a lot of active women into trouble, because they take in more calories than their body is actually burning off." —Kelly Devine Rickert, MS, RD, CSSD, LDN (www.kellydevinenutrition .com), certified specialist in sports nutrition

DON'T OVERDO GELS, BARS, BLOCKS, AND DRINKS

"Just because pros use sports drinks, bars, and gels doesn't mean that you need them too. In fact, if you're trying to lose weight, water and real food can work for most training sessions." —Heather Mangieri, MS, RD, CSSD

DEFINE YOUR GOAL

Is your goal to run a marathon or to lose weight? If you really want to accomplish a marathon, great—just don't expect to lose weight. If you are running to lose pounds, you're going to need to focus on more than running to win at losing.

FAT HABIT #97

When I have a pig-out, I just exercise it off. —KELLY P.

If you believe you can down that bottle of soda or an extra brownie, or even enjoy a fast-food pig-out because you'll just "exercise it off," you're going to have to have an Olympian's training program to keep up with the calories.

The hardest concept to get across to people is that for all the hard work you do in your workout, it takes only a few bites to replenish all those calories that you huffed and puffed away.

SLIM SOLUTION

If you stick with our meal plans (see Chapter 7), you won't be eating foods that cause your blood sugar levels to spike, and they won't trigger the "eat more" responses in your brain, so you'll be less likely to want to pig out.

If you do think you can burn off extra calories with exercise, be sure to keep tabs on the calories of what it is you're considering eating; then think about how much time, sweat, and energy you're going to use to burn them off.

WHAT IT TAKES TO BURN OFF . . .

Here's how much time you have to spend to burn off your favorite foods and beverages*:

EAT OR DRINK THIS . . .	BURN IT OFF WITH . . .
1 chocolate bar (220 calories)	½ hour of hiking or 20 minutes of jumping rope
A 20-ounce bottle of soda (250 calories)	1 hour of house cleaning or 15 minutes of fast swimming
1 plain bagel (350 calories)	1 hour of yard work or 50 minutes of hiking
1 mixed alcoholic drink (400 calories)	1 hour of doubles tennis or 45 minutes of singles tennis
1 slice homemade fruit pie (440 calories)	½ hour of jumping rope or 2½ hours of cleaning
1 fast-food hamburger (500 calories)	1¾ hour of yoga or walking
1 chocolate of Frappuccino (550 calories)	45 minutes of moderate running or fast cycling
1 fast-food shake (560 calories)	1 hour of fast cycling or 2¼ hours of yoga
1 individual pan cheese pizza (620 calories)	1 hour of hard cardio gym exercise or 2¼ hours of walking

*Calculations based on a 150-lb. person.

FAT HABIT #98

I walk . . . isn't that enough? —CASEY R.

Walking is great—it's what our bodies are genetically designed for—but when you're struggling to lose pounds, you'll probably need to change your routine up a bit. And if you want a body that's tight and toned and helps to keep you flexible and fit as you age, you need to add resistance training and flexibility to the mix. (See Fat Habit #92 "I don't lift weights because I don't want to look like a man," for the ACSM's physical activity guidelines.)

However, our golden rule for fitness is to do what you love, because you're more likely to do it. While walking is a great low-intensity exercise, it burns only about 100 calories a mile, and it will take you forty-five minutes to an hour to walk 3½ miles or burn off about 350 calories. Activities that use both your upper and lower body, like jogging, rowing, swimming, or circuit training, can burn two to three times as many calories per minute as walking.

SLIM SOLUTIONS

If you love to walk and have a routine, that's great. But if you want to amp up the fitness and calorie burn-off of your walking workout, here's what you can do:

DO INTERVALS

Interval training can be a great way to get more out of your walking workout. You can do all kinds of intervals by increasing your pace for shorter periods of time, followed by easy recovery walking. This type of training is also great when you combine walking with functional body-weight moves to strengthen muscles.

Warm up for ten minutes; then pick up the pace for two minutes; stop and perform one minute of resistance moves (air squats, burpees, sit-ups, lunges, push-ups, triceps dips on a bench, step-ups); then recover with three minutes of easy walking. Repeat this routine four or five times; then cool down.

HIT THE HILLS

Walking uphill significantly boosts the calories burned by more than twice the calories per minute. Stairs will do the same thing too! For part of your walk, try to find an incline and spend half of your walk on the incline.

PICK UP THE PACE

The easiest way to get more out of a walk is to walk faster. A race walker burns almost as many calories per minute as someone who's jogging. Keep a log and track how long it takes you to do a specific course; repeat that course once a week and see if you can beat your times.

USE YOUR ARMS

If you pump your arms when you walk, you'll start using muscles in your upper body and burning more calories. Bend your elbows at a 90-degree angle and swing from your shoulders like a pendulum in quick swift movements. You can also invest in walking poles to get even more of a workout.

GO ON A HIKE

Julie always says hiking is just walking done in the woods, but hiking burns significantly more calories per minute than walking on flat, smooth pavement. When you're on a trail, you use the smaller muscles of your feet, ankles, and legs to stabilize on uneven terrain, and hikes usually have a lot of ups and downs. It's a great way to take in some nature and improve your fitness at the same time.

PACK ON A FEW POUNDS

No, we don't want you to gain weight to burn more calories on your walk, but using a weighted vest can significantly boost the number of calories you burn during your walk. Add a 10-pound weighted vest and your calories burned per minute will take a hike upward. You can use a hydration pack filled with water to get a sense of what a weighted vest would feel like.

STRENGTH-TRAINING RESOURCES

If you're new to strength training, here are a few websites we find helpful.

BodyBuilding.com—www.bodybuilding.com
CrossFit Journal—http://journal.crossfit.com
Muscle & Fitness Hers—www.muscleandfitnesshers.com

FAT HABIT #99

I hate to sweat. . . . It makes me feel so dirty. —JANE K.

Don't you know that sweat is fat crying? Julie tells herself this at almost every CrossFit workout when she's literally dripping in her fat cells' tears. The benefit of exercise that is so intense that you can't stop sweating is that it boosts your metabolism long after you've stopped exercising. Just like how your body works hard to stay warm in the cold, it also burns extra calories to cool you off when you're sweating.

A recent study found that one forty-five-minute high-intensity cycling session resulted in an elevation in metabolism for fourteen-plus hours. The subjects' bodies were essentially burning more calories at rest compared with days when they did not exercise. Research shows that the higher the intensity of the workout, the more your metabolism will be elevated afterward. Walking, however, doesn't provide enough oomph to get your engine really revving.

SLIM SOLUTIONS

If sweating really keeps you from working out, here are some ideas of ways to get fit that are sweat-free:

TRY STRENGTH TRAINING

Hitting the gym to do a weight-lifting routine won't raise your heart rate enough to make you sweat. Focus on doing exercises that target the major muscle groups of your lower and upper body, and do this at least two or three times a week.

HIT THE H_2O

Swimming, water aerobics, or other activities in a pool or body of water are great for those who don't want to feel sweaty. Swimming is a total-body conditioner and burns lots of calories per minute because it uses all of the major muscles in your upper and lower body, but being in water, you can't feel your perspiration.

TRY FLEXIBILITY AND RANGE-OF-MOTION EXERCISES

Stretching in front of the TV, at a park, or whenever you have a few moments is a great way to make sure you maintain or improve the mobility of your joints.

WALK

Walking won't make you break out in a sweat, but it will help you burn some additional calories. It's so easy and convenient; do it as much as you can.

CLEAN AND DO YARD WORK

These activities also count toward your activity workout minutes, but they're not taxing enough to really make you start sweating.

FAT HABIT #100

I don't like to exercise . . . and didn't exercise to lose weight. Why would I start now? —SUSAN S.

Losing weight is a relatively easy proposition. Eat fewer calories than your body requires and you lose weight. Keeping it off, however, is another story. That's why everyone says diets don't work, and so many people are yo-yo dieters, losing and gaining the same 5, 10, 20, or more pounds over and over again.

Researchers now know that to keep weight from creeping back up, one of the main strategies is daily physical activity. In fact, people who have lost weight require the most exercise to keep that weight off—about an hour a day, most days of the week.

SLIM SOLUTIONS

If exercise isn't your thing, we get it. There are other approaches to get your body to burn more calories to help prevent weight gain. Also, if you're not going to commit to a fitness routine, we suggest that you weigh yourself daily, as successful dieters who do so are the least likely to regain lost pounds. There's something about stepping on a scale that makes you more diligent about what you eat.

A NON-EXERCISE ANSWER

Often, those who don't like to exercise don't mind other ways to move their body, like walking on the beach, riding a bike in a park, walking a dog, dancing, or playing a team sport.

The best thing you can do is find out what you might like that involves moving your body for sixty minutes a day. If you like dogs, maybe being a dog walker is a solution.

Most people spend nearly nine and a half hours a day, or sixty-five hours a week, being completely sedentary, so standing up at least once every half hour will add to calories burned, and add years to your life. A recent study published in the *Archives of Internal Medicine* found that adults who sat the most (more than eleven hours per day) were 40 percent more likely to die over the course of the four-year study, compared with those who sat less than four hours a day. Sitting was found to increase the risk of death, regardless of how fit the subjects were, and their exercise habits.

Ramp up your non-exercise activity thermogenesis (called NEAT), which is the calories burned from movements not considered exercise. Research from the Mayo Clinic reported that obese individuals burn about 350 fewer NEAT calories than lean individuals. Overweight individuals often plant themselves like a flower and are less likely to get up and add minutes of movement to their day.

ADD SOME NEAT-NESS TO YOUR DAY

Fidget, tap your fingers, move your legs as you sit, chew gum, stand up a lot, pace, squat down to pick things up off the floor, stand while sending e-mails or talking on the phone. For a seat at your desk, use an exercise ball instead of a chair. Take the stairs, manually change the channels on the TV, carry your groceries, park farther away than you need to whenever you're parking. All these little changes will help burn extra calories.

Another way to boost your movement during the day is to wear a pedometer. A study by researchers at Stanford University, published in the *Journal of the American Medical Association*, found that pedometer wearers increased their daily steps from the number they took when they didn't wear a pedometer by an average of two thousand. That's about a 25-percent increase in steps per day—about a mile, or an extra 100 calories incinerated—without even trying! Just wearing a pedometer will make you conscious of how much—or how little—you move during the day.

Bottom line: You're not a geranium . . . so don't "plant" yourself during the day. Getting off your bum frequently may be more important than doing a specific workout every day.

9

APPETITE FOR HEALTH'S SLIM SOLUTIONS RECIPES

FAT HABIT #101

I don't know where to find healthy recipes that taste great. I've had so many that just bombed when I tried them. —DONNA B.

As nutritionists, we're always on the lookout for great-tasting recipes with a nutritional profile that won't blow your entire calorie budget. If your primary recipe source is Pinterest, Paula Deen, or cans of cream of mushroom soup, you probably need Appetite for Health's recipe rehab.

You can always adapt unhealthy recipes by swapping out ingredients, but the results are never guaranteed. The best bet is to start with recipes that are designed to pump up the flavor but without all the fat and calories.

SLIM SOLUTION

Great taste and good nutrition shouldn't be mutually exclusive. There's nothing more delicious than fresh, wholesome ingredients cooked to perfection with minimal fuss. These recipes are where we put all of our nutrition and healthy eating guidelines into practice.

Our recipes are easy to make and include world flavors, including lightened-up Mexican meals, easy Asian dishes, spicy Indian soups and main dishes, Mediterranean favorites, and a few all-American classics too (read: mac 'n' cheese and meat loaf).

Each recipe has been developed to provide the nutrition you need to be healthy. We've also designed our recipes with satiety in mind—these meals will keep you fuller longer, because they are protein- and fiber-rich. Each is made with our go-to ingredients, like chicken, turkey, salmon, and lean red meats; hearty veggies and leafy greens; whole grains; low-fat dairy products; and healthy, fat-burning fats like nuts, seeds, avocados, and vegetable oils. We liberally use fresh and dried herbs and spices to punch up the flavor—not the calories.

All of the recipes are less than 400 calories per serving and can be easily incorporated into our 1,600-calorie-a-day meal plans in Chapter 7. In fact, many of the recipes in the following pages are already part of our meal plan solutions.

Enjoy!

BREAKFASTS

SPINACH, MUSHROOM, AND LEEK FRITTATA

6 large eggs
2 egg whites
½ cup skim milk
Pinch of salt and pepper
1 tablespoon olive oil
1 garlic clove, minced

4 cups fresh baby spinach (about half of a 10-ounce package of
spinach), coarsely chopped
1 cup sliced white button mushrooms
1 leek, cleaned and sliced (can substitute 1 cup diced white onions
or green onions)
3 ounces reduced-fat Gruyère cheese, grated (Jarlsberg, Parmesan,
Swiss, feta, or goat cheese can also be used)

■ Preheat broiler.

■ In a medium bowl, whisk eggs and add in milk, half of the cheese, and salt and pepper. In a 12-inch ovenproof nonstick pan, heat olive oil and add garlic and cook for 1 to 2 minutes over medium heat. Add spinach, mushrooms, and leek and cook until vegetables are tender, about 5 minutes. Season with additional salt and pepper, if desired.

■ Remove vegetables from pan and add to egg mixture. Clean pan and spray with nonstick cooking spray. Return pan to medium heat, add egg mixture to the pan, and let the bottom of the eggs set, about 4 to 5 minutes. Sprinkle the remaining cheese on top of the frittata. Broil for 2 to 3 minutes until slightly puffed, golden, and firm throughout. Let frittata sit for 5 minutes before cutting into wedges.

SERVES 4 (2 WEDGES EACH)
Calories 270; Fat 14g (4g sat); Protein 19g; Carb 9g; Fiber 3g; Chol 345mg; Sodium 370mg

SWISS-STYLE MUESLI

1½ cups old-fashioned oats
½ cup chopped dried fruit (e.g., apricots, dates, raisins, dried
cranberries)
1 cup nonfat milk
1 cup nonfat plain Greek yogurt
1 tablespoon coconut flakes
1 medium apple, chopped

1 tablespoon slivered almonds, chopped walnuts, or chopped
  pistachios
1 tablespoon honey
1 tablespoon orange juice

▪ Mix oats with all other ingredients in a bowl. Chill in refrigerator for at least 1 hour before eating, or overnight.

SERVES 4
Calories 260; Fat 4g (1g sat); Protein 13g; Carb 48g; Fiber 5g; Chol 1mg; Sodium 60mg

PROTEIN PANCAKES

2 eggs (or 1 egg plus 2 whites)
1 small banana, mashed (great use for overripe bananas,
  or substitute pureed pumpkin or sweet potato)
1 tablespoon peanut or almond butter
Pinch of cinnamon, if desired
¼ teaspoon vanilla or almond extract, if desired

▪ In a mixing bowl add the eggs to the mashed banana and mix well. Stir in nut butter and cinnamon or extract. In a nonstick skillet on medium heat, lightly oil the pan or use nonstick cooking spray. Pour a large spoonful of batter into the hot pan and cook until browned on one side (3 to 4 minutes or more); flip and brown the other side for another 2 to 3 minutes.

▪ Serve with ½ cup nonfat Greek yogurt and fresh berries on top with a drizzle of honey or agave.

SERVES 1 (3 MEDIUM-SIZE PANCAKES)
Calories 300; Fat 17g (4g sat); Protein 17g; Carb 24g; Fiber 3.5g; Chol 430mg; Sodium 208mg

BREAKFAST EGG SANDWICH

1 whole-wheat English muffin
1 cooked egg

1 slice low-fat (2 percent) American cheese
½ cup arugula
1 ¼-inch-slice tomato
1 tablespoon light mayo

■ Cook egg and toast whole-wheat English muffin. Assemble egg, cheese, arugula, and tomato slice onto English muffin. Top with the mayo.

SERVES 1
Calories 316; Fat 12.6g (3.6g sat); Protein 19g; Carb 38g; Fiber 7; Chol 175mg; Sodium 772mg

STRAWBERRY-BANANA YOGURT PARFAIT

1 cup nonfat plain Greek yogurt
¼ cup sliced strawberries
½ medium banana
½ cup old-fashioned oats

■ In a glass or bowl, alternately layer strawberries, yogurt, oats, and banana. Garnish with strawberry halves and oats. Chill or serve immediately.

SERVES 1
Calories 320; Fat 3g (.5g sat); Protein 26g; Carb 48g; Fiber 6g; Chol 0mg; Sodium 85mg

SCRAMBLED-EGG BREAKFAST BURRITO

1 whole-wheat flour tortilla (130 calories or less)
1 large egg
Dash salt
Dash ground pepper
¼ teaspoon extra virgin olive oil
2 tablespoons grated cheddar or pepper-jack cheese
¼ cup salsa

1 tablespoon sour cream

1–2 tablespoons chopped green chilies (optional)

■ Preheat oven to 350°F. Wrap tortilla in foil and heat in the oven for 5 to 10 minutes, or layer between paper towels and microwave for 20 seconds. Blend egg, salt, and pepper in a medium bowl with a fork until blended. Heat oil in a 10-inch nonstick skillet over medium-low heat. Add chilies, if desired, and cook, stirring, for 1 minute. Add egg mixture, stirring slowly until soft, fluffy curds form (about 1½ to 2½ minutes).

■ Serve eggs on tortilla; top with cheese, sour cream, and salsa.

SERVES 1

Calories 370; Fat 15g (6g sat); Protein 20g; Carb 39g; Fiber 7g; Chol 232mg; Sodium 780mg

LUNCHES AND DINNERS

BAJA-STYLE FISH TACOS

1½ teaspoons olive oil

2 tablespoons lime juice, divided

1½ teaspoons sugar

1½ teaspoons red wine vinegar

¼ teaspoon kosher salt

½ avocado, diced

½ small red pepper, diced

½ small red onion, minced*

3 rings fresh pineapple, diced

2 teaspoons chili powder

½ teaspoon ground cumin

½ teaspoon onion powder

Salt and pepper to taste

1¼ pounds halibut or other firm white fish

8 6-inch flour or whole-wheat tortillas

- In a small bowl, combine olive oil and half of the lime juice with sugar, vinegar, and salt and mix well. Add avocado, red pepper, onion, and pineapple. Cover and refrigerate for 30 to 60 minutes to let flavors combine.

- Create a marinade for the fish with lime juice, chili powder, cumin, onion powder, and salt and pepper. Rub on fillets; cover and let stand 30 minutes before grilling.

- When ready to eat, heat grill to medium, about 375°F. Brush grill grate with oil; grill fish with some marinade still clinging until just opaque in center, about 5 minutes per side. Grill tortillas until slightly charred on both sides. To serve, divide fish evenly among tortillas and top with pineapple salsa. Wrap and eat.

If raw onion is a bit too strong, soak the minced onion in cold water and drain before adding it to mixture.

SERVES 4 (2 TACOS PER SERVING)
Calories 370; Fat 10g (2g sat); Protein 28 g; Carb 44g; Fiber 3g; Chol 54mg; Sodium 610mg

CRANBERRY-TURKEY PANINI

½ teaspoon olive oil
2 tablespoons jellied cranberry sauce
2 slices whole-grain bread
1 ounce reduced-fat cheddar cheese
1½ ounces low-sodium deli turkey
½ medium apple, sliced thin
½ teaspoon olive oil

- Heat panini press or small nonstick skillet brushed with oil over medium heat.

- Spread cranberry sauce on one side of each bread slice. On one slice layer cheese, turkey, and apple. Top with second slice of bread, cranberry side down.

■ Place sandwich on heated pan. Close press and cook until golden brown and toasty, about 5 to 8 minutes. If using skillet, top sandwich with heavy plate wrapped in foil. Press down to flatten. Cook approximately 3 minutes on first side; flip and continue cooking on second side until golden brown and toasty, about 3 minutes longer.

SERVES I

Calories 380; Fat 12g (5g sat); Protein 23g; Carb 45g; Fiber 6g; Chol 35mg; Sodium 663 mg

SALMON MELT FLORENTINE

2 ounces ready-to-eat salmon (from can or pouch)
2 teaspoons reduced-fat mayonnaise
1 whole-wheat English muffin, toasted
¼ cup fresh baby spinach
2 slices tomato
1 tablespoon reduced-fat shredded cheddar cheese

■ Preheat oven or toaster oven to broil. Combine salmon and mayo. Spread evenly on muffin halves. Divide spinach between two halves. Place a tomato slice on each muffin. Sprinkle cheese evenly over tomatoes. Place under broiler until cheese melts.

SERVES I

Calories 325; Fat 14g (4g sat); Protein 22g; Carb 28g; Fiber 3g; Chol 57mg; Sodium 385mg

ASIAN PORK TENDERLOIN RICE BOWL

2 tablespoons olive oil
1 pound lean pork tenderloin, cut into bite-size pieces
¼ cup sugar
2 tablespoons tamari
6-ounce can pineapple juice
¼ cup white vinegar

3 cloves garlic, minced or grated
2 teaspoons grated fresh ginger
Dash cayenne pepper
1½ tablespoons cornstarch dissolved into 3 tablespoons cold water
1½ cups steamed broccoli
1 green onion, sliced (optional)
2 cups cooked brown rice

■ Heat oil in medium skillet over medium heat. Add lean pork tenderloin and sauté until golden brown. While pork cooks, in a small saucepan combine next seven ingredients and heat gently. Add cornstarch mixture, stirring until thickened. Pour sauce over pork, add broccoli, and stir to coat. Sprinkle green onion over top. Serve on top of rice.

SERVES 4

Calories 365; Fat 11g (3g sat); Protein 23g; Carb 44g; Fiber 3g; Chol 60mg; Sodium 565mg

CHILI-TOPPED BAKED POTATO

4 medium russet potatoes, scrubbed
2 teaspoons olive oil
2 tablespoons chopped onion
¼ cup chopped red pepper
½ pound 95 percent lean ground beef
½ 15.5-ounce can black beans, rinsed and drained
½ 14.5-ounce can diced tomatoes in sauce, not drained
½ 8-ounce can tomato sauce
1½ teaspoons chili powder
¼ cup reduced-fat shredded cheddar

■ Preheat oven to 400°F.
■ Using a fork, poke several holes in the potatoes. Once oven is heated, place potatoes on a baking sheet in oven and bake until a butter knife slides in easily, about 45 minutes to 1 hour.

▨ While potatoes are cooking, heat oil in medium-size sauce pot over medium heat. Add onion and pepper and cook, stirring often, until almost tender. Add beef and cook, stirring often to break up meat, until no pink remains. Add next four ingredients. Mix well. Reduce heat to low, cover, and simmer 30 minutes, stirring occasionally.

▨ Remove potatoes from oven and, with a fork, poke an X on top. Push in on ends of potato to open it up. Spoon chili onto each potato and sprinkle with cheese.

SERVES 4

Calories 338; Fat 7g (3g sat); Protein 21g; Carb 49g; Fiber 7g; Chol 40mg; Sodium 228mg

CRUNCHY MACARONI TUNA SALAD

¾ cup whole-grain elbow macaroni
5-ounce can water-packed tuna, drained
3 tablespoons reduced-fat mayonnaise
1 cup baby peas (canned or frozen)
¼ teaspoon garlic powder
1 medium stalk celery, chopped
2 tablespoons minced red onion*
Dash kosher salt
Dash pepper

▨ Cook macaroni according to package directions. While macaroni cooks, combine remaining ingredients. Drain pasta and, while still hot, add tuna mixture and mix well.

*If raw onion is a bit too strong, soak the minced onion in cold water and drain before adding it to mixture.

SERVES 2

Calories 345; Fat 9g (2g sat); Protein 25g; Carb 41g; Fiber 7g; Chol 45mg; Sodium 581mg

PISTACHIO-CRUSTED SALMON

1/3 cup shelled pistachios
1 cup basil leaves, loosely packed
2 garlic cloves
2 tablespoons olive oil
¼ cup fresh-squeezed lemon or lime juice
Salt and pepper to taste
4 salmon fillets (about 4 ounces each), skin on

■ Process first five ingredients in food processor, until ingredients are thoroughly chopped and blended. Add salt and pepper to taste. Using your hands, press the pistachio paste over the top (nonskin side) of each salmon fillet, forming a crust. Grill or bake (400°F) with salmon skin-side down until the fish becomes flaky and is opaque throughout.

SERVES 4
Calories 335; Fat 23g (3g sat); Protein 26g; Carb 6g; Fiber 2g; Chol 60mg; Sodium 150mg

MEDITERRANEAN-STYLE PASTA WITH CHICKEN

2 teaspoons extra virgin olive oil
1 large garlic clove, minced
½ cup onion, chopped
Salt and pepper to taste
⅓ cup sun-dried tomatoes, chopped
¼ cup low-sodium chicken broth
2 tablespoons kalamata olives, pitted and sliced
3 ounces dry short pasta (e.g., farfalle or gemelli)
1 roasted or grilled skinless chicken breast (or 4 ounces cooked
    chicken breast)
1 ounce feta cheese (about ¼ cup)
1 cup cherry or grape tomatoes, sliced
½ cup fresh basil leaves, chopped

▪ In a skillet over medium heat, add olive oil; then add garlic and onion, salt and pepper. Cook until onion is tender. Add sun-dried tomatoes and chicken broth, and simmer until the liquid is reduced. Stir in olives, reduce heat, and keep warm.

▪ In a pot, bring water to a boil, add pasta, and cook according to package directions. Drain pasta, and add it and diced chicken to the skillet and toss. Sprinkle with feta cheese and stir in fresh tomatoes; top with chopped fresh basil.

▪ Serve immediately.

SERVES 2

Calories 390; Fat 14g (3g sat); Protein 23g; Carb 46g; Fiber 5g; Chol 43mg; Sodium 560mg

ROAST BEEF WRAP

1 8-inch whole-wheat tortilla
1 tablespoon horseradish spread (recipe below)
2 ounces thinly sliced low-sodium roast beef
1 ounce reduced-fat cheddar cheese
2 medium slices tomato
½ cup chopped romaine lettuce

Horseradish Spread

¼ cup nonfat plain Greek yogurt
2 teaspoons prepared horseradish
Dash kosher salt
Dash black pepper
Dash garlic powder

▪ Combine all five ingredients for the horseradish spread; mix well and refrigerate until ready to use. To assemble, spread tortilla with horseradish spread. Lay roast beef on top. Lay cheddar down the middle of the wrap, followed by tomato and lettuce. Roll up, slice in half, and enjoy.

SERVES I

Calories 330; Fat 12g (6g sat); Protein 27g; Carb 27g; Fiber 4g; Chol 55mg; Sodium 750mg

SWEDISH MEATBALLS

Courtesy of SkinnyTaste.com (www.skinnytaste.com)

1 teaspoon olive oil
1 small onion, minced
1 clove garlic, minced
1 celery stalk, minced
¼ cup minced parsley
1 pound 93 percent lean ground beef
1 egg
¼ cup bread crumbs
Salt and pepper to taste
½ teaspoon allspice
2 cups reduced-sodium beef stock
2 ounces light cream cheese

■ In a large, deep sauté pan, heat oil on medium, add onion and garlic, and sauté until onions are translucent, about 4 to 5 minutes. Add celery and parsley and cook until soft, about 3 to 4 more minutes. Let cool a few minutes.

■ In a large bowl, combine beef, egg, onion mixture, bread crumbs, salt, pepper, and allspice. Mix well and form meatballs with your hands, ⅛ cup each (fill ¼ cup, then divide the meat in half).

■ Add beef stock to the pan and bring to a boil. Reduce heat to medium-low and slowly drop meatballs into the broth. Cover and cook about 20 minutes. Remove the meatballs with a slotted spoon and set aside in a serving dish. Strain the stock, add to blender with cream cheese, and pulse until smooth. Return to pan and simmer a few minutes to thicken; then pour over meatballs. Garnish with parsley and serve over noodles, or with toothpicks if you want to set these out as an appetizer.

MAKES 20–22 MEATBALLS

SERVES 4 (5 MEATBALLS WITH GRAVY)

Calories 215; Fat 10g (5g sat); Protein 25g; Carb 8.5g; Fiber 1g; Chol 80mg; Sodium 345mg

GRILLED CHICKEN BRUSCHETTA

Courtesy of SkinnyTaste.com (www.skinnytaste.com)

¼ cup chopped red onion
1 tablespoon extra virgin olive oil
1 tablespoon balsamic vinegar
Kosher salt and fresh cracked pepper to taste
3 medium vine-ripe tomatoes
2 small cloves garlic, minced
2 tablespoons fresh basil leaves, chopped
3 ounces part-skim mozzarella, diced
1¼ pounds (8 thin-sliced) chicken cutlets

■ Combine onion, olive oil, balsamic vinegar, salt, and pepper. Set aside for a few minutes. Chop tomatoes and place in a large bowl. Combine with garlic, basil, onion-balsamic combo, and additional salt and pepper to taste. Let sit at least 10 minutes or as long as overnight. Toss in the cheese when ready to serve.

■ Season chicken with salt and pepper. Grill chicken cutlets indoors or on an outdoor grill; top with bruschetta and serve immediately.

SERVES 4
Calories 240; Fat 8.5g (2g sat); Protein 32.5g; Carb 7g; Fiber 1.5g; Chol 63mg; Sodium 183mg

BROCCOLI MAC 'N' CHEESE

¾ pound broccoli crowns, cut into bite-size florets
2 teaspoons olive oil
1½ cups whole-wheat elbow macaroni
2 tablespoons canola oil
2 tablespoons flour
½ cup skim milk
6 ounces (about ⅓ pound) reduced-fat American cheese, shredded
*   or cubed*

■ Heat oven to 400°F.

■ Spread broccoli on a large baking pan. Drizzle with olive oil. Use hands to mix around, making sure broccoli is evenly coated with oil. Roast 20 minutes, shaking pan halfway through to stir broccoli around a bit. When done, remove from oven and reduce heat to 350°F.

■ While broccoli roasts, cook macaroni according to package directions. Drain, rinse with warm water, and set aside.

■ Heat canola oil in a medium saucepan over medium heat. Add flour and cook, stirring, about 1 minute. Whisk in milk. Simmer over medium heat until thickened. Remove from heat and add American cheese; whisk until smooth. Add drained macaroni and stir well to evenly coat macaroni. Pour into 2-quart casserole dish. Gently stir in broccoli. Cover.

■ Bake for 15 minutes covered. Remove the lid/cover and bake for another 15 minutes, or until bubbling and browned.

SERVES 4

Calories 370; Fat 17g (5g sat); Protein 20g; Carb 40g; Fiber 5g; Chol 25mg; Sodium 755mg

CAJUN MEAT LOAF

½ cup ketchup
1 teaspoon hot sauce, such as Tabasco (more or less to desired taste)
1 pound lean ground beef (93–95 percent lean)
¾ cup oats
½ teaspoon crushed red pepper
1 teaspoon cumin
1 teaspoon onion powder
1 egg
1 (5.5-ounce) can of low-sodium tomato juice
¼ cup freshly grated Romano cheese
Dash of salt
Dash of pepper

- Preheat oven to 350°F.
- In a small bowl, combine ketchup and hot sauce. Set aside.
- In a medium bowl, combine remaining ingredients and mix well. Place in an 8×4-inch loaf pan. Place meat loaf in preheated oven. Bake 30 minutes. Pour ketchup mixture over; spread to cover evenly if necessary. Bake an additional 30 minutes.

SERVES 4

Calories 280; Fat 9g (4g sat); Protein 28g; Carb 20g; Fiber 2g; Chol 110mg; Sodium 625mg

CITRUS SALAD WITH GRILLED CHICKEN

12 ounces skinless, boneless chicken breasts, grilled or roasted, sliced
8 cups mixed greens
½ cup parsley, roughly chopped
1 cup thinly sliced fennel
2 cups sliced cucumber

Dressing

2 large oranges
¼ cup freshly squeezed lemon juice
4 teaspoons honey
1 teaspoon Dijon mustard
¼ teaspoon kosher salt
Freshly ground black pepper to taste
¼ cup extra virgin olive oil

- Slice off the peel and pith from the oranges and cut between the membranes to remove the segments; set aside. In large bowl, combine lemon juice, honey, mustard, salt, pepper, and olive oil. Whisk well to combine.
- To the large bowl with prepared dressing, add greens, parsley, orange segments, fennel, and cucumber; toss gently. Divide salad on four serving plates and top with sliced grilled or roasted chicken.

SERVES 4
Calories 365; Fat 16.7g (2.5g sat); Protein 27g; Carb 28g; Fiber 6g; Chol 66mg; Sodium 387mg

MUFFIN-TIN TURKEY MEAT LOAF

1¼ pounds ground turkey (light meat, no skin)
1 cup finely chopped onions
½ cup finely chopped red or green bell pepper
½ cup finely diced carrots
¼ cup Parmesan or Romano cheese, grated
2 garlic cloves, minced
1 cup button or cremini mushrooms, finely chopped
¼ teaspoon salt
½ teaspoon black pepper
½ teaspoon oregano
⅓ cup finely chopped fresh parsley
⅓ cup ketchup
2 teaspoons Worcestershire sauce
1 cup plain or Italian-style bread crumbs (or make with 2 slices
 stale bread in food processor)
2 eggs, lightly beaten

▪ Preheat oven to 375°F. Lightly spray a muffin pan with cooking spray.

▪ Combine all ingredients in a large bowl, saving half of the ketchup and half of the Worcestershire sauce, and mix well with your hands, being careful not to overmix. Divide the turkey mixture equally among the muffin cups. Mix remaining ketchup and Worcestershire sauce together for a glaze and add to mini loaves halfway through cooking.

▪ Bake for 20 to 25 minutes, or until a toothpick inserted into the center of the meat loaf is clean.

▪ Let meat loaves stand 5 minutes before serving.

SERVES 6 (2 LOAVES PER SERVING)
Calories 250; Fat 5.5g (2g sat); Protein 31g; Carb 21g; Fiber 3g; Chol 115mg; Sodium 725mg

SALMON BURGERS WITH LEMON SAUCE

*1 14-ounce can reduced-sodium Alaskan salmon,
   drained and flaked*
1 egg, beaten
½ cup chopped spring onions
¼ cup chopped fresh parsley
¼ cup minced red bell pepper
1 cup bread crumbs
2 tablespoons lemon juice
Dash of hot pepper sauce, if desired
Salt and pepper to taste
¼ teaspoon smoked paprika
1 garlic clove, minced
*4 whole-wheat thin-style or calorie-reduced buns (80 to 100
   calories per bun)*

Lemon Sauce

3 tablespoons reduced-fat mayonnaise
2 teaspoons lemon juice

■ Mix together salmon with next ten ingredients and form four large patties.

■ Spray a nonstick skillet with nonstick cooking spray and preheat over medium to medium-high heat. Cook salmon patties 4 minutes per side. Whisk mayonnaise with lemon juice to make lemon sauce and season with black pepper and paprika, if desired.

■ Serve patties with lemon sauce on reduced-calorie toasted whole-wheat buns with lettuce and tomato slices, mustard, and other condiments.

SERVES 4
Calories 310; Fat 14g (2.5g sat); Protein 21g; Carb 24g; Fiber 2g; Chol 80mg; Sodium 785mg

SHRIMP AND CORN CHOWDER

3 large baking potatoes, peeled and cubed
2 cups chicken stock
1 cup skim milk
¼ teaspoon kosher salt
¼ teaspoon pepper
1½ cups fresh or frozen corn kernels (or one 11-ounce can,
  drained)
½ pound small shrimp, peeled and deveined
2 slices reduced-sodium turkey "bacon," cooked and crumbled

■ Place potatoes in a large microwave-safe bowl. Microwave on high 5 minutes, stirring halfway through heating. Stir in stock and milk, salt, and pepper. Microwave 10 more minutes, stirring halfway through heating. With a slotted spoon remove about ⅓ of potatoes and set aside.

■ With an immersion blender or electric mixer mash together remaining potatoes and liquid until creamy. Place liquid mixture in a large saucepan and heat over medium-high heat. Stir in remaining potatoes, along with corn and shrimp. Continue heating, stirring often, until shrimp is no longer pink, 5 to 10 minutes. Serve topped with turkey bacon.

SERVES 4

Calories 345; Fat 3g (1g sat); Protein 20g; Carb 61g; Fiber 6g; Chol 75mg; Sodium 755mg

TACO SALAD

½ onion, diced
3 garlic cloves, minced
1 pound lean ground beef (93–95 percent lean)
½ head iceberg lettuce, shredded (about 4 cups)
2 medium tomatoes, diced
1 avocado, diced

½ cup salsa
4 ounces baked tortilla chips, slightly crumbled
⅓ cup fresh cilantro, chopped

Taco Seasoning

>*Use ½ packet store-bought beef taco seasoning, or*
>*1 tablespoon chili powder; ½ teaspoon each salt, pepper, garlic*
>   *powder, and ground cumin; and ¼ teaspoon each crushed red*
>   *pepper and oregano*

■ On medium to medium-high heat, in nonstick skillet sprayed with nonstick cooking spray, sauté onion and garlic for 2 to 3 minutes until fragrant. Add ground beef to onion and garlic, and add taco seasoning to skillet. Stir and continue to brown beef. When beef is well cooked, pour off grease.

■ On a platter, layer lettuce, seasoned ground beef, diced tomatoes, avocado, salsa, and crumbled tortilla chips. Garnish dish with fresh cilantro.

MAKES 4 SERVINGS
Calories 400; Fat 24g (6g sat); Protein 31g; Carb 30g; Fiber 8g; Chol 70mg; Sodium 575mg

APPLE-AND-WALNUT-STUFFED CHICKEN BREASTS

1½ cups whole-wheat bread cubes
½ cup reduced-sodium chicken stock or broth
1 tablespoon butter
1 cup peeled, cored, and chopped green apple
½ cup chopped onion
3 tablespoons pure maple syrup
½ cup chopped walnuts
1 tablespoon chopped fresh rosemary (plus additional for topping
  chicken, if desired)
Salt and freshly ground pepper to taste
4 small boneless, skinless chicken breasts

■ Preheat oven to 375°F. Place bread on a baking sheet and cook for 15 minutes or until crisp. Place in a large bowl and pour stock over top; let stand for 5 minutes.

■ Melt butter in a large skillet. Add apple and onion; cook over medium heat for 10 minutes, stirring frequently, until very soft. Stir in maple syrup. Add apple mixture, walnuts, and herbs to bread cubes and mix well; season to taste with salt and pepper. Cut a slit in each chicken breast to form a large pocket. Fill with stuffing mixture and place in a shallow baking dish. Season with salt, pepper, and rosemary; cook for 1 hour or until chicken is cooked through.

SERVES 4

Calories 310; Fat 15g (3g sat); Protein 23g; Carb 23g; Fiber 3.5g; Chol 55mg; Sodium 490mg

INDIAN GARBANZO SOUP

1 (16-ounce) package dry garbanzo beans
1 (48-ounce) container reduced-sodium chicken broth
4 cloves garlic, chopped
3 carrots, peeled and sliced
1 large onion, chopped
1½ teaspoons each ground cumin and ground coriander
1 teaspoon garam masala (available in the spice section of most
* grocery stores)*

■ Soak or quick-soak beans according to package directions; drain well, then place in a large saucepan with broth, garlic, carrots, and onion. Bring to a boil; reduce heat and simmer, covered, for 1 hour or until beans are very tender.

■ Puree in a blender or food processor or with an immersion blender until very smooth. Place back in pan and add seasonings; cook for 10 minutes more.

SERVES 8
Calories 230; Fat 3.5g (0g sat); Protein 17g; Carb 35g; Fiber 6.5g; Chol 3.5mg; Sodium 450mg

MEXICAN QUINOA AND BLACK BEAN SALAD

1 cup quinoa
1⅓ cups vegetable stock
1 teaspoon chili powder
1 teaspoon each ground cumin and dried oregano
½ cup diced red bell pepper
2 green onions, sliced
1 (15-ounce) can black beans, rinsed and drained
Snipped fresh cilantro
1 grilled or roasted chicken breast, sliced

Dressing

¼ cup extra virgin olive oil
3 tablespoons lime juice
1 teaspoon sugar
¼ teaspoon salt

▪ Rinse quinoa in a fine mesh sieve and drain well. Place in a medium saucepan with stock and seasonings and bring to a boil. Reduce heat and simmer, covered, for 12 minutes. Remove from heat and let stand for 10 minutes. Let cool; then stir in pepper, onions, and beans.

▪ Stir together all dressing ingredients in a small bowl and then stir into salad. Add chicken. Cover and chill for at least 1 hour.

SERVES 4
Calories 380; Fat 14g (2g sat); Protein 20g; Carb 43g; Fiber 7g; Chol 19mg; Sodium 665mg

SHRIMP, FETA, AND COUSCOUS

2 cups couscous or quinoa
½ onion, chopped
1 tablespoon extra virgin olive oil
1 can (28 ounces) reduced-sodium Italian-style plum tomatoes,
  drained
¼ cup dry white wine
2 teaspoons dried oregano
¾ pound raw shrimp, shelled and deveined
3 ounces feta cheese, crumbled (about ¾ cup)
2 tablespoons fresh parsley, chopped

■ Prepare couscous or quinoa according to package directions and keep warm.

■ In large nonstick skillet on medium heat, sauté onion in olive oil until onion turns translucent (about 3 minutes). Add tomatoes, wine, and oregano. Reduce heat to low and simmer for about 5 minutes. Add shrimp and cook for 3 to 5 minutes, stirring until shrimp are pink. Sprinkle with feta cheese.

■ Serve over warm couscous or quinoa and top with fresh parsley.

SERVES 4
Calories 315; Fat 9g (4g sat); Protein 25g; Carb 35g; Fiber 5g; Chol 200mg; Sodium 700mg

OVEN-FRIED CHICKEN TENDERS

1 pound chicken tenders
¾ cup all-purpose flour
½ teaspoon salt
1 teaspoon black pepper
½ teaspoon paprika
Pinch cayenne or chili pepper
2 eggs, slightly beaten

2 tablespoons water

1½ cups whole-wheat panko bread crumbs (use seasoned bread crumbs, if desired)

■ Preheat the oven to 425°F. Line a jelly pan with aluminum foil and place a baking rack on top of the foil. Spray the baking rack with nonstick cooking spray and place each tender on the rack.

■ On a plate, combine flour, ½ each salt and black pepper, paprika, and cayenne or chili pepper. In a small bowl, whisk together 2 eggs with 2 tablespoons water. On another plate, spread panko bread crumbs.

■ Pat chicken tenders dry and coat each tender with flour; then dip each tender into the egg wash and then roll in the panko crust. Cook for approximately 12 to 15 minutes, or until chicken tender reaches 165°F.

Note: If you don't have a baking rack, cook tenders for 10 minutes on aluminum foil–lined pan, then turn and cook another 2 to 5 minutes.

SERVES 4

Calories 335; Fat 4.5g (.5g sat); Protein 32g; Carb 42g; Fiber 4g; Chol 170mg; Sodium 800mg

CHICKEN TIKKA KEBABS OVER JASMINE RICE

1¼ pounds boneless, skinless chicken breasts (cut into strips)
Bamboo skewers, soaked in water 30 minutes
1 to 2 fresh lemons, halved

Tikka Seasoning

2 teaspoons each: turmeric, dried cilantro leaves, ground ginger, ground cumin, ground coriander, chili powder, and garlic salt

■ Preheat an outdoor grill to medium-high heat, about 375°F. Spray grill grate with nonstick cooking spray.

■ Stir together all tikka seasonings in a small bowl. Cut chicken into ⅛-inch-thick diagonally cut strips and sprinkle liberally on both sides with tikka seasoning. Thread onto bamboo skewers.

■ Cook on a grill over medium heat, turning while cooking for about 7 minutes total. Squeeze lemons over chicken during the last 2 minutes of cooking. Serve with basmati rice seasoned with saffron, parsley, and fresh-squeezed lemon juice.

SERVES 4

Calories 135; Fat 4.5g (.5g sat); Protein 22g; Carb 1g; Fiber 1g; Chol 60mg; Sodium 700mg

STRAWBERRY CHEESECAKE BITES

Courtesy of the California Strawberry Commission (www.calstrawberry.com)

1 package (8 ounces) reduced-fat cream cheese (Neufchâtel cheese), softened
⅓ cup powdered sugar
2 teaspoons lemon juice
½ teaspoon grated lemon peel
20 (just over 1 pound) whole, stemmed California strawberries
8 graham cracker squares, finely crushed (about ⅔ cup)

■ In mixer bowl, beat together cream cheese, sugar, lemon juice, and lemon peel until smooth and creamy; set aside. Using a paring knife or small melon baller, partially hollow out top of strawberries to a depth of ¾ inch. Gently fill each with 1 tablespoon cream-cheese mixture.

■ Roll tops into graham cracker crumbs. Arrange on serving platter.

■ For chocolate cheesecake variation, melt ½ cup semisweet chocolate morsels as package directs; stir into one 8-ounce package cream cheese (softened). Add ⅓ cup powdered sugar and ½ teaspoon vanilla extract.

◼ Proceed as recipe directs, rolling filled strawberries into finely crushed graham crackers or chocolate wafer cookies.

◼ Tip: To prepare recipe ahead of time, fill strawberries with cream-cheese mixture; cover and refrigerate up to 6 hours. Roll in graham cracker crumbs just before serving.

SERVES 20

Calories 40; Fat 1.5g (1.0g sat); Protein 1g; Carb 5g; Fiber <1g; Chol 5mg; Sodium 585mg

CLASSIC SHEPHERD'S PIE MADE SKINNY

Courtesy of SkinnyTaste.com (www.skinnytaste.com)

1 pound ground turkey
1½ teaspoons olive oil
1½ cups onions, diced
1 cup carrots, diced
1 cup celery, diced
1 tablespoon fresh garlic, minced
1 teaspoon dried thyme
3 tablespoons all-purpose flour
2 tablespoons tomato paste
1 (14.5-ounce) can diced tomatoes, undrained
1 cup reduced-sodium chicken broth
½ cup red wine
1 tablespoon Worcestershire sauce
2 teaspoons Dijon or yellow mustard
1 cup frozen green peas

Topping

7 cups frozen hash brown potatoes, not thawed
3 tablespoons reduced-fat butter or Smart Balance Light,
*   melted, or olive oil or canola oil cooking spray*
Salt and pepper, to taste

- Preheat oven to 400°F.

- Coat a 12×9- or 13×9-inch baking dish with nonstick cooking spray. Set aside. In a large nonstick pan, brown ground turkey over medium-high heat, about 8 to 10 minutes. Pour turkey into a colander and drain all the fat. Blot with paper towels. Set aside.

- In same pan, heat 1½ teaspoons olive oil over medium heat. Add onions, carrots, and celery and sauté until soft, about 5 minutes. Add garlic and thyme and cook for 1 minute. Stir in flour and tomato paste; cook for 1 minute. Stir in tomatoes, broth, wine, Worcestershire, and mustard. Bring to a boil; reduce heat to medium-low and stir in cooked ground turkey and peas. Pour filling into baking dish and place on baking sheet.

- For the topping: Arrange frozen hash browns on top of filling. Lightly press the potatoes down to keep them mounded. Drizzle melted butter all over top of potatoes, or spray olive oil or canola oil cooking spray over the top. Sprinkle with a little salt and pepper to taste.

- Place casserole in oven and bake for 45 to 50 minutes, until potatoes are golden brown.

- Let pie cool for 15 minutes to set before serving.

SERVES 8

Calories 538; Fat 30g (<.5g sat); Protein 25g; Carb 46g; Fiber 5g; Chol 30mg; Sodium 473mg

CHICKEN POT PIE SKINNYFIED

Courtesy of SkinnyTaste.com (www.skinnytaste.com)

3 cups reduced-sodium chicken broth
1½ cups onions, chopped
1 cup potato, peeled and cubed (½-inch cubes)

1 cup sweet potato, peeled and cubed (½-inch cubes)
1 cup carrots, peeled and chopped
1 cup celery, sliced
1 pound chicken breasts (boneless, skinless), cut into bite-size
*   pieces*
1½ cups frozen peas (not defrosted)
1½ cup reduced-fat milk
½ cup plus 1 tablespoon all-purpose flour
2 tablespoons fresh thyme, chopped, or 1 teaspoon dried
¼ teaspoon salt
¼ teaspoon fresh-ground black pepper
1 package Pillsbury Golden Layers flaky biscuits (100 calories for
*   each biscuit)*

▪ Preheat oven to 350°F. In a large pan, add the chicken broth and bring to a boil. Stir in the onions, potato, sweet potato, carrots, and celery. Bring back to a boil, reduce heat, and cover. Simmer for 6 minutes. Add the chicken pieces and frozen peas, breaking them up. Bring back to a boil, turn the heat to simmer, cover, and cook for 5 minutes.

▪ Place a colander into a large bowl. Pour the chicken, vegetables, and broth into the colander. Add the strained broth back to the pan. Set aside the chicken and vegetables.

▪ In a separate small bowl, add the flour. Gradually add the milk to the flour, stirring with a whisk, until well blended. Increase the heat to medium with the broth. Stir in the milk/flour mixture with a whisk. Cook for 5 minutes, or until thickened. Stir often. Add back the chicken and vegetables, along with the thyme, salt, and pepper. Mix well.

▪ Coat an 11×7-inch baking dish with cooking spray and pour in the chicken stew. Open the package of biscuits, separate them, and place on top of the chicken stew, lining them evenly. Place the pie on a foil-lined baking sheet and bake for 14 minutes, until the biscuits are golden brown.

■ To serve, spoon into each bowl and top with one biscuit. There will be two extra biscuits for whoever desires.

SERVES 8

Calories 266; Fat 6g (<.5g sat); Protein 20g; Carb 38g; Fiber 4g; Chol 32mg; Sodium 653mg

ACKNOWLEDGMENTS

WITHOUT THE UNWAVERING SUPPORT OF OUR REAL SKINNY TEAM, including our fans, clients, colleagues, and publishing partners, this book would not have been possible. Thank you to Sara Carder for your enthusiasm from the start, and your extraordinary editing to bring the job to completion. We would also like to thank our agent, Jane Dystel, for her experience and expert insights.

This book could not have been written without our professional colleagues who graciously provided us with their time, best practices, feedback, and encouragement; we could not have done it without you. Thank you for your input and for helping to move our profession forward.

I (KATHERINE) would like to express my gratitude to the many people who saw me through this book. First and foremost, I would like to thank my mother, Eileen, and sister, Christine, whose love and support helped to make this book, and all that I do, possible.

I also wish to thank my dear friends Firouzeh Murray, Lauren Cantor, Julie Levitt, Cindy Nelson, Eric Newman, and Chris Led-with. I am forever grateful for your love, support, laughter, and willingness to allow me to ramble from time to time. Last but not least, to my four-legged, goofy pals Ollie and Jack: Thank you for waiting just one more minute. . . . You guys are the best!

I (JULIE) am especially grateful for my family, who graciously puts up with my unpredictable work schedule and time away from home. To Craig, my rock, who always believes in me—even when I doubt myself. And especially, to my mom, sisters, nieces, and nephew, your steady presence in my life provides me with the ability to be my best.

REFERENCES AND
SUGGESTED READING

CHAPTER I

Centers for Disease Control. Current depression among adults in the United States, *MMWR.* 2010; 59(38): 1229–35.

Del Coso, et al. Dose response effects of a caffeine-containing energy drink on muscle performance: a repeated measures design, *J Int Soc Sports Nutr.* 2012; 9: 21.

Deshmukh-Taskar PR, Nicklas TA, O'Neil CE, Keast DR, Radcliffe JD, Cho S. The relationship of breakfast skipping and type of breakfast consumption with nutrient intake and weight status in children and adolescents: the National Health and Nutrition Examination Survey 1999–2006. *J Am Diet Assoc.* June 2010; 110(6): 869–78.

Epel ES, Needham, BL, et al. Trajectories of change in obesity and symptoms of depression: the CARDIA Study. *Am J Public Health.* June 2010; 100(6): 1040–46.

Fowler SP, Williams K, Resendez RG, Hunt KJ, Hazuda HP, Stern MP. Fueling the obesity epidemic? Artificially sweetened beverage use and long-term weight gain. *Obesity.* 2008; 16: 1894–1900.

Gold MS, Graham NA, Cocores JA, Nixon SJ. Food addiction? *J Addict Med.* 2009; 3: 42–45.

Hill AJ. Does dieting make you fat? *Br J Nutr.* 2004; 92(1).

Hill J, Thompson H, and Wyatt H. Weight maintenance: What's missing? *J. Am. Diet. Assoc.* 2005; 105: S63–S66.

Mattes RD, Popkin BM. Nonnutritive sweetener consumption in humans: effects on appetite and food intake and their putative mechanisms. *Am J Clin Nutr.* 2009; 89: 1–14.

Parsons TJ, Power C, Logan S, Summerbell CD. Childhood predictors of adult obesity: a systematic review. *Int J Obesity.* 1999; 23: S1–S107.

Pelchat ML. Food addiction in humans. *J Nutr.* 2009; 139: 620–622.

Piers LS, Soares MJ, McCormack LM, O'Dea K. Is there evidence for an age-related reduction in metabolic rate? *J Appl Phys.* December 1998; 85(6): 2196–204.

Strychar I, Lavoie ME, Messier L, Karelis AD, Doucet E, Prud'homme D, et al. Anthropometric, metabolic, psychosocial, and dietary characteristics of overweight/obese postmenopausal women with a history of weight cycling. *J Am Diet Assoc.* 2009; 109(4): 718–24.

Vermunt SH, Pasman WJ, Schaafsma G, Kardinaal AF. Effects of sugar intake on body weight: a review. *Obes Rev.* May 2003; 4(2): 91–99.

Whitaker RC, Wright JA, Pepe MS, Seidel KD, Dietz WH. Predicting obesity in young adulthood from childhood and parental obesity. *NEJM.* 1997; 337: 869–73.

Yang Q. Gain weight by "going diet"? Artificial sweeteners and the neurobiology of sugar cravings. *Yale J Biol Med.* June 2010; 83(2): 101–108.

Zhang C, Rexrode KM, van Dam RM, Li TY, Hu FB. Abdominal obesity and the risk of all cause, cardiovascular, and cancer mortality. sixteen years of follow-up in U.S. women. *Circulation.* Apr 1, 2008; 117(13): 1658–67.

CHAPTER 2

Berge JM, Larson N, et al. Are parents of young children practicing healthy nutrition and physical activity behaviors? *Pediatrics.* 2011; 4: 881–87.

Bove CF, Sobal J. Body weight relationships in early marriage: weight relevance, weight comparisons, and weight talk. *Appetite.* 201; 57(3): 729–42.

Christakis NA, Fowler JH. Social contagion theory: examining dynamic social networks and human behavior. *Stat Med.* 2012 Jun 18. doi: 10.1002/sim.5408. [E-pub ahead of print]

Cunningham SA, Vaquera E, Maturo CC, Narayan KM. Is there evidence that friends influence body weight? A systematic review of empirical research. *Soc Sci Med.* 2012; 75(7): 1175–83. E-pub 2012 Jun 19.

Gorin A, Phelan S, Tate D, Sherwood N, Jeffery R, Wing RR. Involving support partners in obesity treatment. *Journal of Consulting and Clinical Psychology.* 2005; 73(2): 341–43.

Herring SJ, Rose MZ, Skouteris H, Oken E. Optimizing weight gain in pregnancy to prevent obesity in women and children. *Diabetes Obes Metab.* 2012; 14(3): 195–203.

Hruschka DJ, Brewis AA, Wutich A, Morin B. Shared norms and their explanation for the social clustering of obesity. *Am J Public Health.* 2011; 101 Suppl 1: S295–300.

Shoham DA, Tong L, Lamberson PJ, et al. An actor-based model of social network influence on adolescent body size, screen time, and playing sports. *PLoS One.* 2012; 7(6): e39795. E-pub 2012 Jun 29.

Sobal J, Hanson KL, Frongillo EA. Gender, ethnicity, marital status, and body weight in the United States. *Obesity.* 2009; 17(12): 2223–31.

Tiffin R, Arnoult M. The demand for a healthy diet: estimating the almost ideal demand system with infrequency of purchase. *Eur Rev Agric Econ.* 2010; 37(4) 501–21.

CHAPTER 3

American Cancer Society. www.cancer.org

American College of Sports Medicine. www.acsm.org

American Diabetes Association. www.diabetes.org

American Heart Association. www.heart.org

American Institute for Cancer Research. www.aicr.org

Celiac Disease Foundation. www.celiac.org

Celiac Facts and Figures. www.celiaccentral.org/celiac-disease/facts-and-figures

Center for Science in the Public Interest. www.cspinet.org

Leidy HJ, Tang M, Armstrong CLH, Martin CB, Cambell WW. The effects of consuming frequent, higher protein meals on appetite and satiety during weight loss in overweight/obese men. *Obesity.* 2011; 19: 818–24.

Office of Dietary Supplements (National Institutes of Health)—www.dietary-supplements.info.nih.gov

Prevalence of Overweight and Obsesity. www.cdc.gov/nchs/data/hestat/overweight/overweight_adult.htm

Ratliff J, Leite JO, de Ogburn R, Puglisi MJ, VanHeest J, Fernandez ML. Consuming eggs for breakfast influences plasma glucose and ghrelin, while reducing energy intake during the next 24 hours in adult men. *Nutrition Research.* 2010; 30: 96–103.

Sumithran P, Prendergast LA, Delbridge E, Purcell K, Shulkes A, Kriketos A, Proietto J. Long-term persistence of hormonal adaptations to weight loss. *N Engl J Med.* 2011; 365: 1597–1604.

St-Onge MP, Bosarge A. Weight-loss diet that includes consumption of medium-chain triacylglycerol oil leads to a greater rate of weight and fat mass loss than does olive oil. *Am J Clin Nutr.* March 2008; 87(3): 621–26.

Tufts University Health & Nutrition Letter. www.tuftshealthletter.com

Young LR, Nestle M. Portion sizes and obesity: responses of fast-food companies. *J Public Health Policy.* July 2007; 28(2): 238–48.

CHAPTER 4

Chandon P, Hutchinson JW, Bradlow ET, Young SH. Does in-store marketing work? Effects of the number and position of shelf facings on brand attention and evaluation at the point of purchase. *J Mark.* 2009; 73: 1–17.

Cohen DA. Obesity and the built environment: changes in environmental cues cause energy imbalances. *Int J Obes.* December 2008; 32 Suppl 7: S137–42.

Cohen DA, Babey SH. Contextual influences on eating behaviors: heuristic processing and dietary choices. *Obes Rev.* 2012; May 3. doi: 10.1111/j.1467-789X.2012.01001.

Cohen DA, Bhatia R. Nutrition standards for away-from-home foods in the USA. *Obes Rev.* July 2012; 13(7): 618–29.

Cohen DA, Finch BK, Bower A. Collective efficacy and obesity: the potential influence of social factors on health. *Social Science & Medicine.* 2006; 62(3): 769–78.

Guthrie JF, Lin BH, Frazao E. Role of food prepared away from home in the American diet, 1977–78 versus 1994–96: changes and consequences. *J Nutr Educ Behav.* 2002; 34: 140–50.

Levy AS, Fein SB. Consumers' ability to perform tasks using nutrition labels. *J Nutr Educ.* 1998; 30: 210–17.

Sorensen H. Long tail media in the store. *J Advert Res.* 2008; 48: 329–38.

Sutherland LA, Kaley LA, Fischer L. Guiding stars: the effect of a nutrition navigation program on consumer purchases at the supermarket. *Am J Clin Nutr.* 2010; doi: 10.3945/ajcn.2010.28450C.

Todd JE, Mancino L, Lin BH. The impact of food away from home on adult diet quality. Economic Research Report no. 90. 2010. Washington, DC: USDA Economic Research Service; available at www.ers .usda.gov/ publications/err90/err90.pdf.

Wu WW, Sturm R. What's on the menu? A review of the energy and nutritional content of U.S. chain restaurant menus. *Public Health Nutr.* 2012; 11: 1–10.

CHAPTER 5

Cornell CE, Rodin J, Weingarten H. Stimulus-induced eating when satiated. *Physiology & Behavior.* 1989; 45(4): 695–704.

Deshpandé R, Wansink B. "Out of sight, out of mind": the impact of household stockpiling on usage rates. *Marketing Letters.* January 1994; 5:1; 91–100.

Hu FB, Li TY, Colditz GA, Willet WC, Manson JE. Television watching and other sedentary behaviors in relation to risk of obesity and Type 2 Diabetes Mellitus in women. *JAMA.* 2003; 289(14): 1785–91.

Keith SW, Reddin DT, et al. Putative contributors to the secular increase in obesity: exploring the roads less traveled. *International Journal of Obesity.* 2006; (30): 585–94.

Scheibehenne B, Todd PM, Wansink B, Dining in the dark: the importance of visual cues for food consumption and satiety. *Appetite.* 2010; 55:3: 710–13.

St.-Onge M, Roberts AL, Chen J, Kellerman M, O'Keeffe M, Jones P. Short sleep duration increases energy intakes but does not change energy expenditure in normal-weight individuals. *Am J Clin Nutr.* August 2011; (2): 410–16.

Van Ittersum K, Wansink B. Plate size and color suggestibility: the Delboeuf Illusion's bias on serving and eating behavior. *Journal of Consumer Research.* August 2012. [E-pub ahead of print.]

Wansink B, Painter JE, North J. Bottomless bowls: why visual cues of portion size may influence intake. *Obes Research.* 2005; 13: 93–100.

Wansink B, Cheny MM. Super bowls: serving bowl size and food consumption. *JAMA.* April 2005; 293(14): 1727–28.

Wansink B. Environmental factors that increase the food intake and consumption volume of unknowing consumers. *Annu. Rev. Nutr.* 2004; 24: 455–79.

CHAPTER 6

Bellisle F, Drewnowski A, Anderson GH, Westerterp-Plantenga M, Martin CK. Sweetness, satiation, and satiety. *J Nutr.* June 2012; 142(6): 1149S–54S.

Cassady BA, Considine RV, Mattes RD. Beverage consumption, appetite, and energy intake: what did you expect? *Am J Clin Nutr.* 2012; 95(3): 587–93.

Ello-Martin JA, Ledikwe JH, Rolls BJ. The influence of food portion size and energy density on energy intake: implications for weight management. *Am J Clin Nutr.* July 2005; 82(1 Suppl): 236S–241S.

Leidy HJ, Apolzan JW, Mattes RD, Campbell WW. Food form and portion size affect postprandial appetite sensations and hormonal responses in healthy, nonobese, older adults. *Obesity.* February 2010; 18(2): 293–99.

National Restaurant Association. Facts at a Glance. www.restaurant.org/research/facts/

Physicians Committee for Responsible Medicine Airport Review 2011. (Online: www.pcrm.org/health/reports/2011-airport-food-review.)

Piernas C, Popkin BM. Increased portion sizes from energy-dense foods affect total energy intake at eating occasions in U.S. children and adolescents: patterns and trends by age group and sociodemographic characteristics, 1977–2006. *Am J Clin Nutr.* November 2011; 94(5): 1324–32.

Racette SB, Weiss EP, Schechtman KB, Steger-May K, Villareal DT, Obert KA, Holloszy, JO. Influence of weekend lifestyle patterns on body weight. *Obesity.* 2008; 168: 1826–1830.

Wu HW, Strum R. What's on the menu? A review of the energy and nutritional content of U.S. chain restaurant menus. RAND Corporation. March 2012 DOI: http://dx.doi.org/10.1017/S136898001200122X.

CHAPTER 8

Bartlett JD, Close GL, MacLaren DP, Gregson W, Drust B, Morton JP. High-intensity interval running is perceived to be more enjoyable than moderate-intensity continuous exercise: implications for exercise adherence. *J Sports Sci.* 2011. 29: 547–53.

Bauman AE, Reis RS, Sallis JF, Wells JC, Loos RJ, Martin BW. Correlates of physical activity: why are some people physically active and others not? *Lancet.* 2012 Jul 21; 380(9838): 258–71.

Bravata DM, Smith-Spangler C, Sundaram V, et al. Using pedometers to increase physical activity and improve health: a systematic review. *JAMA.* 2007; 298(19): 2296–304.

Britton KA, Lee IM, Wang L, et al. Physical activity and the risk of becoming overweight or obese in middle-aged and older women. *Obesity.* 2012; 20(5): 1096–103. doi: 10.1038/oby.2011.359. [E-pub 2011 Dec 22.]

Brooks GA, Butte NF, Rand WM, Flatt JP, Caballero B. Chronicle of the Institute of Medicine physical activity recommendation: how a physical activity recommendation came to be among dietary recommendations. *Am J Clin Nutr.* 2004; 79(5): 921S–930S.

Garber CE, Blissmer B, Deschenes MR, et al. American College of Sports Medicine position stand. Quantity and quality of exercise for developing and maintaining cardiorespiratory, musculoskeletal, and neuromotor fitness in apparently healthy adults: guidance for prescribing exercise. *Med Sci Sports Exerc.* 2011; 43(7): 1334–59.

Knab AM, Shanely RA, Corbin KD, Jin F, Sha W, Nieman DC. A 45-minute vigorous exercise bout increases metabolic rate for 14 hours. *Med Sci Sports Exerc.* 2011; 43(9): 1643–48.

McCullough LE, Eng SM, Bradshaw PT, et al. Fat or fit: The joint effects of physical activity, weight gain, and body size on breast cancer risk. *Cancer.* 2012 Jun 25. doi: 10.1002/cncr.27433. [E-pub ahead of print.]

van der Ploeg HP, Chey T, Korda RJ, Banks E, Bauman A. Sitting time and all-cause mortality risk in Australian adults. *Arch Intern Med.* 2012 Mar 26; 172(6): 494–500.

INDEX

If you enjoyed this book, visit

www.tarcherbooks.com

and sign up for Tarcher's e-newsletter to receive
special offers, giveaway promotions, and
information on hot upcoming releases.

TARCHER
PENGUIN

Great Lives Begin with Great Ideas

New at **www.tarcherbooks.com**
and **www.penguin.com/tarchertalks:**

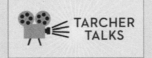

Tarcher Talks, an online video series featuring
interviews with bestselling authors on everything from creativity and prosperity to 2012
and Freemasonry.

If you would like to place a bulk order
of this book, call 1-800-847-5515.